Seniors on the Move

Renate Rikkers

Amherst Keep Fit Association, Inc.

Human Kinetics Publishers, Inc.

Champaign, Illinois

Library of Congress Cataloging-in-Publication Data

Rikkers, Renate, 1941-
    Seniors on the move.

    Bibliography: p.
    Includes index.
    1. Physical fitness for the aged—Study and
teaching.   I. Title.
GV482.6.R55   1986   613.7'0240565   85-24846
ISBN 0-87322-040-4

Developmental Editor: Susan Wilmoth, PhD
Production Director: Ernie Noa
Typesetter: Sandra Meier
Copy Editor: Steve Davenport
Text Layout: Janet Davenport
Proofreader: Ann Bruehler
Interior Design: Julie Szamocki
Cover Design and Layout: Jack Davis
Printed by: United Graphics

ISBN 0-87322-040-4

Printed in the United States of America

10 9 8 7 6 5 4 3 2 1

Human Kinetics Publishers, Inc.
Box 5076, Champaign, IL 61820

Seniors on the Move

contents

preface

Thirteen years ago, I made a spontaneous decision to offer a fitness program at our Amherst Senior Center. I had taught adult classes in the community for several years, working with young and middle-aged participants, but began to miss contacts with an older generation. I had left Germany as a young adult, leaving family and older relatives behind, and realized how important these relationships had been to me. The senior center seemed to offer a wonderful opportunity for making older friends and finding some of these contacts I missed.

My offer to come in for a "pep talk" and exercise demonstration was received with interest, but my efforts to involve a dressed-up audience in some simple exercises to music were met with great hesitation. Toward the end of my presentation, just a few people had joined in at their seats, but I did notice a lot of foot-tapping and finger-snapping to the beat of the music. I finished by offering to start a program the following week and encouraged everyone to give it a try.

Only five women came to the first class, in dresses, high heels, and pearls, and I had to wonder whether my idea was a good one. This truly was an experimental endeavor, and I had few materials and guidelines available to help me feel confident. My basic knowledge of the human body and its exercise needs and a sincere interest in being and working with this age group had to guide me.

The first few months were discouraging because participation did not increase by leaps and bounds. I was spoiled by high enrollment in other classes and expected the word to spread like wildfire. Nevertheless, I made a commitment to give this new program a chance. Seeing how much those who came enjoyed this active time together convinced me of the value of such a program and made me believe in its ultimate success. I chose this opportunity to contribute to the community by sharing my enjoyment of an active life with an age group given to sedentary living and "rusting out." In turn I was rewarded with new relationships that greatly enriched my life.

Much has happened since those early beginnings. In time, word did spread and class size grew. The old senior center was torn down and replaced by a wonderful new building with an activity room. We even outgrew this space and moved into a large church hall. We went from meeting once a week to twice a week, and now most everyone would prefer to add a third day.

The participants who attend regularly are approximately 40 well seniors between the ages of 60 and 85. Each class meets for one hour, and everyone agrees that these hours are highlights of the week. Participants eagerly look forward to meeting and always come, regardless of weather. Beyond experiencing the obvious benefits of regular exercise, their reasons for coming are personal and varied. Many live alone and appreciate the socialization these classes offer. They experience renewed vigor and use this energy in many other ways. They develop greater self-confidence and feel in charge of their well-being. Joyful social interaction, laughter, and "playing" again makes everyone feel young and lively. Exercising together creates cohesiveness, promotes cheerful communicating, and releases stress. Many have undergone very noticeable changes in outlook and attitude and have enlarged the scope of their daily lives by opening up to new experiences and ventures.

The exercise boom in this country has become big business. Options for participation exist in abundance for younger generations, and the many benefits derived from exercise are well-documented at this time. However, this national fitness fever has not yet addressed the needs of the older population. Although popular programs and scores of books on the subject of exercise have flooded the country over the past decade, a noticeable void still exists in these areas for our seniors. Fitness, it is implied, is important only for the young. Specific exercise guidelines and a great variety of programs for the young are well-established. If our older population is to be included in this great national wellness movement, much work is left to be done. At this time, the book market can be scanned very quickly, and existing research data is very limited in comparison to what is known about younger age groups.

We all know that the quality of our older years is greatly influenced by how we live. Regular exercise and good nutrition are the cornerstones for maintaining wellness and independence as long as possible. Consistent guidelines for exercise in the "golden years," however, are more difficult to establish than for a young, healthy population. Because of the wide range of physical conditions and states of health, many variables exist, and instructors are understandably wary of teaching an age group about which so little is known. The lack of adequate training opportunities adds to the dilemma and makes it difficult to feel confident. Instructors must rely largely on common sense and a basic belief that exercise is important to overall good health and that the need for movement does not diminish with advancing age.

Teaching would be easier if instructors were given a reliable "recipe" for conducting classes for those over 60. These developments, however, will take time, a fact that should not discourage us from establishing good programs right now. Being as knowledgeable as possible is our first responsibility. Beyond that we have to have the courage to go out and work with this age group, relying on our own good judgment and on the wisdom of those who participate. Instead of looking at exercise merely as a science, it is important to remember that lifelong movement is the most natural and necessary function of the human body. The changes that accompany aging set certain limits when it comes to activity or work, but this is normal and should not discourage us from helping seniors maintain a healthful level of fitness through appropriate programs.

This manual contains much of what I have been privileged to learn while teaching seniors who were willing to experiment, react, and critique. Materials I have compiled are the result of sorting out all that has appealed to my students and has brought about an impressively high level of energy, fitness, and wellness. It will help instructors lead safe, purposeful, and stimulating classes. Emphasis is on the use of exercise to promote physical and mental well-being, on offering a unique opportunity for joyful social interaction, laughter, and physical contact. Suggestions in this manual can result in challenging classes where participants experience significant changes in how they feel, act, and progress. This book is filled with ideas and information, a recipe book for good programs. But without special instructors, these materials will do little to promote a positive attitude toward a more active life at an older age. It is our responsibility as fitness leaders to bring joy and enthusiasm into our classrooms, to be sincere, caring, cheerful, and sensitive in working with older participants. We have the privilege of positively affecting many older lives by encouraging a more active, healthy lifestyle. If instructors bring into the classroom the willingness to do this work with sincere commitment and conviction, this manual will serve its intended purpose.

Renate Rikkers

about the senior models

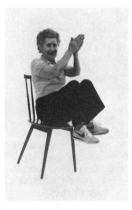
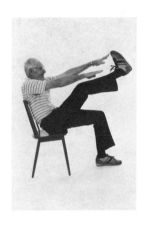
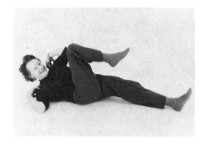

"Both of us love this program and look at it as preventive medicine. We feel good all over at the end of each class. No joint gets by without exercise, and that is so important at our age. It tones muscles and gets blood circulating, makes us feel youthful and energetic. Participating has made us get "hooked" on regular exercise and encourages us to spend 15 minutes every morning with a basic routine to get us ready to start the day. When we are without exercise, we just don't feel as well and feel like we are neglecting ourselves. The program is a challenge that is satisfying to meet, and even though we are usually tired at the end of the class, we have more energy to do other things later. Everyone who is caught in a sedentary lifestyle should participate in some form of exercise to experience how much better one can feel. Exercise keeps us young inside and appreciative of being well."

Polly and Karol Wisnieski are both 71 years old. They grew up on local farms, and for Karol, the family farm continues to provide hard work at planting and harvesting time. He is retired from teaching and administrative work in Public Health but continues to volunteer his time and professional knowledge to public health issues in Amherst. Open heart surgery in 1979 to replace an aorta valve required Polly's retirement from teaching kindergarten. Her cardiologist strongly supports her exercise participation and is impressed with her physical condition, high energy level, and positive attitude. Polly spends time daily with her 96-year-old mother who has suffered several strokes and needs nursing home care. The strong focus of her daily visits is a simple exercise routine she developed to keep her mother as functional as possible (a 101-year-old roommate joins in!). Karol has also had experience in leading exercise: During 6 years of service in the Armed Forces, his daily duties included leading 200 men in their early morning calisthenic workouts!

"This exercise class is definitely one of the high points of my life. It has had a very strong effect on the quality of my life, and I would even venture to say that I believe it is prolonging my life. I have gained so much physical self-confidence in this program and can do things I never believed I could do. At 82, I am proud of being able to keep up with everyone in the class, and many are 20 years younger than I. I have gained the confidence to do new and interesting things, feel good physically and emotionally, and would sum up my feelings by saying that this program is keeping my body toned and my morale high. This is a cohesive, wonderful group of people, and it is very special to spend active time with each other and leave in high spirits each time."

Elizabeth (Libby) Beebe, at 82, is one of the oldest class members and inspires all of us with her energetic participation. She has three sons, eight grandchildren, and a wide circle of friends of all ages. "I love being with young people and believe it is very important to stay current to be an interesting person for younger people to spend time with." To that end, Libby participates in Elderhostel courses, attends lectures and concerts, volunteers as a "god-grandmother" in the Amherst elementary school system, and has been a hospice volunteer for the past 5 years. "I like to challenge myself, and meeting the physical challenges in our program has given me the confidence to seek out challenges in other areas."

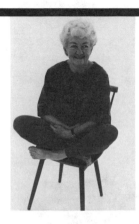 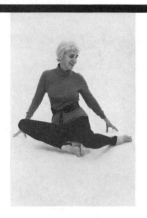 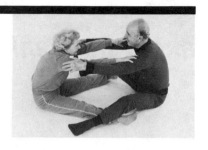

"I think a program such as this is an excellent way to help people steer clear of looking at the aging process in such a negative way. Physical activity breaks down a lot of barriers. Getting people together in a large group for these activities gives everyone a real morale booster. In other social situations it's often easy to feel unwanted, to drift on the perimeter. But here, everyone is equally involved, and there is no competition; each person can feel good about what they are able to do. I love feeling the genuine affection and concern class members have for each other, and appreciate that we are in an atmosphere where physical touching and some hugging happens spontaneously. And I love the opportunity to laugh and let my hair down—it's a real tonic!"

Windy Sayer has kept her age "a deep dark secret" because she is convinced that it prejudices people. It took some doing to have her reveal her age for this introduction: Windy is 72, which is hard to believe. "I am fortunate to have been in good health, and I am a very selective eater. My weight has not changed since college—but it has somehow rearranged itself a bit!" Windy's love for all kinds of dancing keeps her light on her feet and feeling young. She loves gardening, hikes with the Amherst Senior Hikers, and walks as much as possible. Retired from her work as curator of special collections at our local library, she still surrounds herself with books. Windy, too, feels strongly about maintaining friendships with younger people. "They are so much fun to be with, and they stimulate and challenge me mentally."

"I consider this program to be great social recreation. Leaping about with friends is such fun! People make friends with each other and often do other things together. It makes for a friendly and cheerful atmosphere, and it certainly keeps all of us lively, energetic, and healthy."

Anne Inglis will celebrate her 70th birthday soon, and her long legs have made "leaping about" something she has enjoyed all her life. Between raising six children, she took ballet and modern dance classes, and was inspired by belly dancing for many years. With a doctorate in Romance languages, she taught French in her "professional life," but more recently finds herself very busy keeping up with her 11 grandchildren and her love for hiking. Anne leads a committed group of Senior Hikers twice weekly, her long legs setting a brisk pace for easy, intermediate, and advanced outings in all weather. She estimates that the group covers at least 20 miles each week, year around. Anne is convinced that participating in regular exercise has helped her overcome a variety of joint injuries and maintains her in comfort. Anne's activity level is matched by her husband's commitment to running close to 50 miles each week. This couple's retirement is not taking place in rocking chairs!

"This class keeps us alert, active, and healthy. Our lives are very busy, and it's easy to forget how important it is to keep time for exercise. By coming to the class together, we set aside this block of time and truly look forward to it. We love dancing, and exercising to lively music can be just as much fun. These classes are highlights of our week—moving to music in the company of people who become friends over a period of time is special. Beyond providing a good workout for the whole body, it lifts the spirit and makes us feel well all over."

Lois and Harold Smith lead active lives. Lois is a petite 103 lb at 68, "just the same as on the day I married her," says her husband Harold proudly. Lois' life is one of giving and serving—through her church, the Interfaith Council, the League of Women Voters, and to their children, grandchildren, friends, and neighbors. At 70, Harold still holds a part-time professorship in chemistry and continues with consulting research. In his free time, he cuts enough firewood to keep the woodstove going through long winters, walks regularly, and plays golf as often as he can. "Lois really had to cajole me into coming to this class, and it seems that other men don't find it easy to join in—there are so few of us, and that really is unfortunate. I have found this program to be a real delight, and I'm hoping it will make a difference in my golf swing this season!"

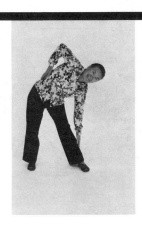 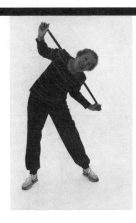 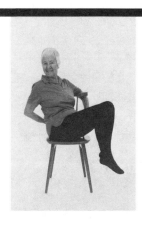

"If I am not physically active, I experience a boring kind of tiredness which really drags me down. Fortunately, it's in my natural makeup to be active, and I have built this class into my regular weekly schedule and love it. It's the kind of exercise I wouldn't take time for on my own, but it is important basic conditioning and works all muscles and joints. I plan to keep up with the program—I know it will keep me limber and feeling youthful in the years ahead."

Eleanor Lachman's 70th birthday is just around the corner, and she attributes her lifelong good health to having inherited good genes. "These genes have kept me healthy and have kept my hair from turning gray!" Eleanor enjoys walking and biking and joins the Senior Hikers at least twice a week. She and her husband Bill have a fascinating and time-consuming retirement hobby: the hybridizing of new varieties of day lilies. Over the years, they have introduced a dozen new varieties, and there is a great deal of work involved. The 4,000 seedlings growing in the Lachman's back yard need care from spring until late fall. To share their interest and enjoyment with others, they travel to day lily lovers' conventions and meetings, always increasing their knowledge and improving their showy display of over 150 varieties of these fast-fading blossoms. "We keep so busy that the word retirement just doesn't seem to apply—and we intend to keep it that way."

"I have always thought of myself as an amateur dancer, and I continue to feel that way in these classes. Next to gardening, this is my favorite activity, and I love coming four mornings a week. It's a wonderful way to get me ready for the day. In addition to being good exercise, it provides great socialization with so many nice people in the community. I consider this program to be a real challenge—it spurs all of us on to be the best we can be and keeps us on our toes."

Carol Burr Cornish is 75 and wears many hats. Her husband, a world-famous golf course architect and author of several books on the subject, has a faithful co-worker in Carol. Avid gardening has replaced her life work as a Jr. Lieutenant in the WAVES and in career counseling for women. Making things grow and prosper is a special source of joy for Carol. Her pride and joy is a nursery where trees are started from seed or seedlings and then potted by the hundreds for the annual garden club sale. Continued mental stimulation is of real importance—"Living in a college community provides this stimulation, and I take full advantage of it."

"I have been coming to this program for over 5 years, and it has been a real boon in many different ways. I can't say enough about the feeling among the people in the group. There is so much real friendship, especially when something difficult happens in someone's life. And I feel limber—none of the stiffness that so many of my older friends complain about. It keeps all the parts moving smoothly, and keeps me in good overall condition for hiking."

Ruth Seymour's hiking boots, backpack, and energetic, purposeful stride make it hard to believe that she is 71 years old. Our class is just a warm-up for long hikes that follow, exploring the many trails in the area. Her husband Stan accompanies her on long walks, and both feel that their good health is due to being outdoors all year around and staying as active as possible. Ruth and Stan are avid square dancers, and they enjoy traveling to many parts of the world. "We are grateful to be in good health so we can enjoy doing so many different things and spend quality time with our three children and four grandchildren. Retirement is a rich and fulfilling time in our lives, and we take good care of ourselves so we can continue to stay well and independent."

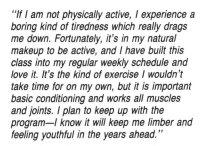

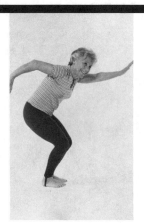

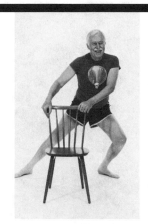

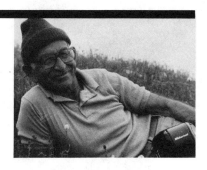

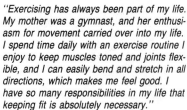

"Exercising has always been part of my life. My mother was a gymnast, and her enthusiasm for movement carried over into my life. I spend time daily with an exercise routine I enjoy to keep muscles toned and joints flexible, and I can easily bend and stretch in all directions, which makes me feel good. I have so many responsibilities in my life that keeping fit is absolutely necessary."

Ruth Dornbush at 60 has more energy than most people half her age. She takes care of two grandchildren every day while the parents work. In addition, she cares for her 90-year-old parents who share the household. Her lifelong passion has been oil painting, and in her sunlit studio she creates beautiful landscapes that turn her house into a gallery and are exhibited as far away as New York. When snow falls, three generations pack up for the slopes: Ruth, her husband Laslo, their children, and grandchildren all enjoy this winter sport and are accomplished and avid downhill skiers. "Life is full and busy, and getting older has not restricted us in our interests and activities. We plan to keep it that way by taking good care of ourselves."

"I have been exercising all my life in one way or another, and to cease now would be disastrous. Physical activity keeps my spirits high, keeps me healthy, mentally stable, and alert. It can be very exhilarating, but I also find it a quieting and calming experience, something I never want to eliminate from my life."

Tom Carhart's military bearing has been part of a long military career. As a fighter pilot, he flew Lockheed Lightnings in Italy during World War II, and before coming to Amherst, he was commander of the Yokota Air Force Base in Japan. His second career was in real estate selling, but such an uneventful earthbound existence made him too restless. He purchased the Silver Eagle, a bright blue hot air balloon, and takes to the skies bright and early every morning with eager passengers in tow. His wife May, recently retired from nursing, mans the chase vehicle and retrieves balloon, pilot, and passengers, greeting them with a bottle of champagne. To keep things lively and interesting, Tom organizes a yearly Teddy Bear Rally on the Amherst town common, inspired by the giant Teddy Bear Rallies in London. He has been collecting Teddy bears from around the world for many years, and when you go up in his balloon, there always is a bear along—with a parachute.

Laslo Dornbush, the photographer for this book, has become a special friend to everyone who modeled. His great sense of humor and relaxed ways made each photo session a special time for all of us. With professional skill, he turned the Amherst Senior Center into a bit of Hollywood, a special experience for those who posed and those who watched. We lost track of the hours he spent in his darkroom, and his commitment to this overwhelming project supported me throughout the writing of this book. "Lazi" brought out the best in each model, and the happy faces smiling at us clearly reflect his warm, personal interaction with each of his subjects.

Laslo is an accomplished nature photographer, and his prize-winning creations are exhibited widely. On weekends, his wife Ruth packs up her easel, Lazi his camera, and they spend many of their happiest and most creative hours in the great outdoors. At 70, Laslo is impressively active. He helps his son-in-law in coaching the Amherst High School ski team. As soon as the first rays of spring sunshine warm the tennis courts, he practices his mean tennis swing and challenges me to lively games. Our personal friendship extends to sharing fabulous meals, hiking, and cross-country skiing. I cannot thank my friend enough for his patient and dependably cheerful attitude throughout our working relationship. Without his expert photography and committed long work hours, this book would not convey the essence and spirit of happy, healthy living in the older years.

1

working with seniors: my personal philosophy

No one wants to be "put on the shelf." All of us, as we look ahead, want to remain active, healthy, respected, and independent members of this society. The trend encouraging elders to take this direction has begun, and we can strongly support these efforts by starting purposeful, creative fitness programs for seniors in communities everywhere.

Statistics show that the older population in this country has grown twice as fast as the rest over the past few decades, and the Bureau of the Census provides surprising figures in its 1984 Current Population Report. In 1950, the over-60 population numbered 18.5 million. By 1980, the group had doubled in size to 36 million. The 1980 figure is expected to increase another 25% by the year 2000, bringing the number of older Americans to 45.5 million, and further growth will continue for at least the first three decades of the next century.

These statistics also show that only 5% of those 65 and over are in nursing homes. The great majority of older persons live independently as members of our communities, and surveys make clear that this is where they want to stay: out of institutions, in their own homes, managing on their own as long as they can.

In 1978, personal health care expenditures for the elderly amounted to almost $50 million or 30% of the total U.S. personal health care bill. Since then, hospital and nursing home costs have continued to soar, forcing state and federal governments to take a hard look at the future. New trends of care are slowly developing, and the focus is on "living better longer"—keeping the elderly out of hospitals and institutions as long as possible. Medical schools across the country are developing stronger focus on courses in geriatric medicine, and health care plans are changing to cover preventive programs and at-home care and support. "Wellness promotion" has become an important concept in the health care field and needs to include our older population so that improved lifestyles will lessen illness and dependence on long-term medical and institutional care.

These slowly developing changes take place at state and federal government levels, but what happens in our communities can strongly support this positive trend. Preventive health care needs of our older population can be addressed through programs that encourage seniors to lead healthier, more active and involved lives. This ever-growing segment of our population has every right to be part of the popular wellness movement, to be informed about nutrition, exercise, and continued good self-care to remain well and independent. Funding and programming directed at the frail elderly need to expand to include those who are well. We as fitness instructors and educators can make a great contribution to these pioneering efforts.

My own attitude toward the process of aging has been strongly influenced by my work and the resulting close personal contacts with many seniors. I no longer view aging as an inevitable process of losses and decline. Instead, I am firmly convinced that we can keep a tight grip on quality living if we so choose.

My older friends have taught me that we should guard against asking too little of ourselves, both physically and mentally, throughout the passing years. To ward off the deterioration we all fear so much, it is essential to keep sufficient physical and mental challenges in our lives. Personal philosophy and attitude strongly determine how we age, and each person has the choice to remain or learn to become active and involved. We have no control over growing older in years, but we can stay fit in body and mind. Many older people decline, not because they run out of potential, but because existing potential is no longer called into play. I strongly believe that it is not so much the passing of years that causes a decline in physical ability, but rather the disuse and lack of continued physical stimulation. I know too many capable people in their 70s and 80s to accept that aging and decline go hand in hand.

Exercise and dietary habits, good health care, continued mental stimulation, and an expectation of well-being will influence how we age. How far we are affected by these factors is an individual choice. No matter what the age, lifestyle can be improved, new doors can be opened, new challenges can be explored,

and new learning can take place. We only have to want it. Sadly, options for participation in physical activities diminish in the older years with the result that physical confidence and ability diminish as well. Depression, a serious and widespread problem among the elderly, contributes to these functional losses by inviting a lethargic, withdrawn lifestyle conducive to giving in to the ailments of the older years. Lack of movement results in decreased ability to move, and unless there is intervention, this negative cycle will continue. Communities and agencies must develop programs and services for seniors to provide this intervention and support a normal, healthy aging process.

The challenges I have offered in our seniors fitness program have been eagerly faced and met by participants. I have learned that there is no reason not to set the same goals for seniors as I do for younger students, giving each person the choice and opportunity to explore his or her individual physical potential. As is true at every age, this potential differs from one person to the next, and it is the instructor's responsibility to support this individual development within the framework of a safe, stimulating classroom setting.

qualities of a good instructor

In teaching, I have been strongly guided by common sense, respect, sensitivity, open-mindedness, and a sense of humor. All these, I have found, are essential ingredients for successfully working with people in general and seniors especially. No amount of specific research data could motivate the seniors I know into regular exercise participation as much as a caring instructor who provides a warm, cheerful, and supportive classroom atmosphere.

common sense and good judgment

Common sense and good judgment are valuable tools to rely on in our teaching. We have become so dependent on data, heart rate charts, and specific scientific guidelines that we have lost confidence in our ability to make good decisions and often forget that we are working with people, individually unique, and in need of personal, sensible guidance. Relying on common sense has given me a solid basis for eliminating inappropriate exercises and activities. Common sense is gained by being knowledgeable, and knowledge supports good decision making. Common sense helps focus on simplicity in movement and purposeful lesson planning, respecting exercise as basic and necessary for lifelong wellness.

respect

Respect for my older students is a strong guide in my work. The most serious mistake we can make is to be condescending in our teaching approach. It is common to "talk down" to older people, often treating them as if they were children. In choosing activities and music, it is crucial to remember that we are working with mature, intelligent adults with extensive life experience. I make every effort not to set myself apart from my students but to work *with* them. I let them know how privileged I feel to learn from them, and how positively their attitudes affect my personal life and my views on aging. Respect for and appreciation of each other is something we all share. Everyone in the group is equally important to the success of the program. We all know this and express it in the way we relate to each other.

awareness and sensitivity

Awareness and sensitivity have helped me see my class not as a whole but as a group of individuals with varying needs, problems, and moods. Facial expressions and body language convey so much, and responding to these signals is important. At times, if I see several frustrated faces in a particular class, it means completely changing the direction I had planned to take. Pain, unwellness, and depression are clearly expressed if we care to look. A personal conversation can lighten a load if we care to help. Sensitivity and awareness mean caring. Coming from the heart, this caring is a genuine concern for each individual with whom we work, making our class time meaningful and enriching.

open-mindedness

Open-mindedness has been important in discarding many preconceived notions about aging. It has been thrilling to discover how physically capable, interesting, and stimulating older persons are. Being open-minded as a group has made experimenting fun, challenging, and successful. Open-mindedness has taught us that many limits are self-inflicted by narrow attitudes and expectations—*not* by physical inability—and that discovering unexpected potential is a great confidence-builder. With an open mind even things that do not go well are fun, just because it is another experience.

good sense of humor

If all this is combined with a good sense of humor, there is little chance of offering an unsuccessful pro-

gram. No matter what my personal day may contain, I never consider the option of not bringing laughter and fun into the classroom. I know that my students do not come just to exercise. They expect our time together to be uplifting and joyful, a time for letting go and having fun. Because we are able to laugh together and to laugh at ourselves, we never feel clumsy, unsuccessful, or incapable. Sharing laughter leaves a warm, happy feeling inside and makes being together special.

The practical tools for teaching are very necessary, of course, as is the theoretical knowledge presently available to us. But the essence of a special program is determined by the human interaction, by the personal relationship between instructor and participants, and by the classroom atmosphere. If trust and caring are the foundation and if teaching comes from the heart, the lack of concrete research guidelines will be much less of a problem. A warm and comfortable classroom atmosphere will enable participants to comment, critique, and guide us in our work, teaching us that the most valuable learning takes place not in research laboratories but in the classroom. Without bringing programs to our communities, no amount of future research data will encourage our seniors to lead more active lives, to take charge of their own well-being, and to get out of rocking chairs and back onto the busy roads of life.

your older students— who are they?

Industrialized societies do not offer great opportunities for purposeful, productive years after retirement. The fragmentation of families has caused the separation of old and young. Intergenerational living has become rare here compared to less industrialized nations where older family members continue to be important contributors, needed and respected by the rest. It is difficult for us who are younger and involved in life and work to imagine this older stage in life when family and work responsibilities almost totally diminish. Gerontology, the study of aging, looks at these complex issues. We do not have to be experts in the field of aging, however, to understand some of the common situations and difficulties older people face. This understanding enables us to make our programs supportive and meaningful group experiences for everyone involved.

In evaluating the effects our fitness program has had on its participants, I am often amazed at how far-reaching they have been. I can best explain this by giving some examples from classroom experience that have been often repeated in slightly different ways over the years I have taught.

Libby joined our class at the age of 80 in a serious state of depression. She had lost her husband several months earlier after nursing him through the last stages of painful bone cancer. When we met, her mental and physical resources were depleted. Their marriage and relationship had been exceptionally close, and Libby had been a very dependent wife. Her identity was closely connected to her husband's position as a faculty member at a local college, even after his retirement. They had traveled together and had an active social life with the college community. His illness came as a grave shock, and the long-term suffering was agony for both.

A friend urged Libby to come along to our class, hoping it would help her make a start at joining life again. She came and went very quietly for several weeks, her posture and facial expressions clearly showing her depressed state. It was obvious that she found it difficult to have fun and join in, and in conversations she made clear that she had to force herself to attend. Her energy level was low, she slept poorly, cried much of the time, and was scared of the future. Several months later, she was a changed person: Her increased vigor showed in her carriage and movements, a smile lit up her face, and she interacted with others in the group. Her depression lifted visibly, and she began to look forward to and thoroughly enjoy our classes. We talked often, and it was heartwarming to realize how much she had been helped at this most difficult time in her life. She developed confidence in her physical abilities, felt much better physically and mentally, and eased her way back into comfortable social relationships.

We were thrilled when Libby announced that she had decided to join an organized tour to New Zealand, something she and her husband had looked forward to doing together. She also became involved in our local hospice organization, helping others to cope with the trauma of terminal illness. Now 82, Libby is one of my star students, a model to all of us, with her high energy level and positive outlook on life and its continued opportunities and challenges.

Several years ago, a neighbor convinced Herb to join us. After his retirement and his wife's death, he had been living alone, puttering around house and yard, struggling with a worsening eye condition. His social contacts were limited, and he spent much of his time alone. The class welcomed him warmly, making him feel comfortable quickly. Class days became important,

providing purpose for his daily walks. Herb walks the 3 miles from his home to our activity center, participates wholeheartedly in our activities, and enjoys staying after class to talk with others.

At first, Herb's failing eyesight concerned me because it was difficult for him to follow my exercise demonstrations. I had to become more aware of the need for clear verbal instructions to help Herb participate safely. During the active part of our class, a class member or I work with him to give him the necessary stability and direction so that he never feels left out.

Through contacts in this class, Herb has also joined the Senior Hikers, a group of avid walkers who meet several times a week. He bought a backpack and hiking boots, and it is a joy to see him march off with this active group for often arduous hikes. Through this program, he has found additional social contacts and the kind of exercise in which he can safely and comfortably participate.

Until a few months ago, however, I did not fully realize the importance of the program in Herb's life. He was scheduled for eye surgery in Boston, and during his last class, we said our good-byes and wished him great results. A few days later, just as I was leaving to teach, Herb called long distance from the hospital. Although he wanted to let me know that he had come through the surgery feeling well, the real reason for his call was to convey how much he would miss our class that morning. He wanted to share with everyone that he was all right and already looked forward to coming back after recuperating. I was touched by his need to make contact with all of us, realizing how much the support and caring of a group can mean to a person who lives alone.

After Joan recovered from a slight stroke, her physician urged her to join us. She had been left with a partial paralysis of her left side, and physical therapy treatments had ended. Joan, having hoped for complete recovery, was discouraged and came to the first class with great hesitation. She had little confidence in her physical abilities and expressed concern about being able to participate. After a long conversation, I urged her to use her good judgment and common sense and do whatever she felt confident and safe with. With her permission, I explained her problems and limitations to everyone, asking for their support and help.

Joan's coordination and ability to participate have improved significantly over a few months. She has developed great confidence in her physical abilities and has learned to work around her problems, rarely needing to sit back and watch. A strong relationship has developed between Joan and another class member who always stands or sits by her side, does partner exercises with her, and offers continual encouragement.

I see these two women go off after class to have a cup of coffee together, obviously enjoying each other's company. The class as a whole is supportive and encouraging and regularly comments on her noticeable improvements. When Joan came to class a few weeks ago in a bright new sweatsuit and running shoes, there were great cheers. Her smile of pride and accomplishment made all of us feel good.

The courage and admirable attitudes displayed by class members have erased the many preconceived notions I once had about aging and adjusting to life's changes. All of us have coping skills, and, with the right attitude, these skills can be put to good use. As an example, Steve is a class member who gives us a real lift twice a week. Formerly an Amherst College ski coach, Steve's life revolved around physical activity. After his retirement, he was diagnosed to have cancer and needed extensive surgery. Several ribs and part of his diaphragm had to be removed. Unfortunately, a nerve to his right leg was damaged during surgery. Because of the extensive muscle atrophy in his right leg, he joined our class on a cane, determined to shape up the rest of his body to compensate for this permanent weakness.

After his surgery, Steve had purchased a rowing machine to work on overall muscle strengthening at home, but walking and balance were still a real problem. With his positive attitude and his high expectations, "Coach Steve" often needed to be discouraged rather than encouraged in his participation. Even though I urged him to progress slowly, the athlete in Steve took over, and he pushed himself to the extreme. On two occasions he fell, his weak leg buckling, unable to support him. Shrugging off his falls, he made it clear that as an avid life-long skier, he has had extensive experience in falling safely. To me, an instructor very concerned about safety and a perfect no-injury record, Steve has been a challenge. Although we have locked horns, I have to respect his strong personality and tremendous willpower. These attributes have helped him cope with life-threatening disease. He assured me that his surgeons, also, had to give in and let him go about things in his own way and that they were highly impressed by his remarkable recovery and physical condition.

There have been no more falls since those early classes, and the cane is in Steve's attic. Through his daily exercise regime, both at home and in our class, this 82-year-old man has developed strong, dependable muscles that help him compensate for the lack of control in his leg. When we skip or run, he walks briskly, his posture proud and erect, his face beaming. He occasionally puts us through our paces by demonstrating his ski team's warm-up drills. Several times a year he waves bon voyage as he and his wife embark on trips to Europe, the Caribbean, and other exciting, exotic places. He comes back tanned, his energy recharged, and we realize that we missed him greatly.

Our older students represent a cross-section of life with its joys and sorrows and have much to teach us. If our hearts and minds are open, we are privileged to affect many lives by offering a supportive, caring, and genuinely warm environment in which to grow, discover new strengths, and build self-confidence. For me, there is not a more satisfying age group with which to work. The love and appreciation I feel from my students is expressed in so many wonderful little ways: a carton of farm-fresh eggs left in my car; a tiny mango tree started from seed; a postcard that says: "I am having a great trip—but miss you and our class!" I am not paid for teaching these classes, but my rewards come in all these special ways. A hug from one of my older students makes my day because it comes right from the heart.

2
you, the instructor: the key to success

While we are young, we spend little time thinking about getting old. It's not a subject with which most of us are comfortable. Young interns observing my classes often express real fear about being with older people. They don't quite know how to interact with them, often because personal emotions interfere. Here they come face to face with the reality that youth does not last, that aging is inevitable. They may, for the first time, give serious thought to their own mortality, which can be a disturbing confrontation. "I am afraid of being with older people," one intern confided. "I think of them as frail and unwell and always expect something terrible to happen while we are together." She agreed that her limited contacts with older persons had probably caused her fears. Her view of old age was one of infirmity, dependence, and senility. But observing our classes and carrying on many lively conversations with participants helped her look at aging in a much more positive light.

evaluating your attitudes

As instructors working with seniors, we need to confront our own attitudes toward aging. What are our fears? How were our attitudes formed, and how will they affect our interactions with older students? How do we envision our personal old age? We live in a society that emphasizes youth and beauty, an attractive body and perfect skin. The normal aging process is viewed with dismay. The appearance of wrinkles can cause panic: If we lose our youthful attractiveness, will people still care about us? Being middle-aged is bad enough, and we wonder what good things old age can possibly have in store. We tend to focus on losses: loss of good health and physical ability, memory, independence, work and family responsibilities. The consequence of all these losses, we conclude, must be years of helplessness and dependence on nursing home care.

It is reassuring to know that only 5% of those over 65 need nursing home care. "Old age" has a very different interpretation now than it did several decades ago. My mother seemed old to me when I was a child and teenager. Today, I find myself in competitive tennis matches with friends in their 60s. Our Amherst Senior Hikers cover many miles each week with backpacks and hiking boots, climbing challenging trails. Many in their 70s and 80s travel extensively, take demanding college courses, and maintain their own homes and property. These are the seniors we can meet in our programs and who can positively affect our views on aging. They are active, open-minded, knowledgeable, interesting, and interested. "I have always been a curious person," one class member said to me on her 80th birthday, "and getting older certainly has not changed me. I will never be too old to learn something new or to enjoy new challenges and experiences." For her 80th birthday, her daughter sent her up in a hot-air balloon, which, incidentally, is owned and operated by a retired Air Force colonel with continued enthusiasm for higher altitudes.

It is a great privilege to have contacts with such people. They teach us so much if we care to learn from their attitudes and experiences. Old age is undeniably a difficult and lonely time for many. Ill health and negative attitudes toward life are problems at any age. It's how we deal with these problems that makes the difference, and here we can learn from and be inspired by our older students' examples.

instructor personality

Just as there is a range of personalities among the seniors we teach, so do instructors' personalities and teaching approaches vary. Each class/instructor combination will be unique. Our individual personality determines the development of our classroom atmosphere. When I visit other programs, I very quickly notice that some feel more comfortable than others. It is easy to detect whether the instructor enjoys his or her work. Genuine enthusiasm for physical activity and sincere enjoyment in working with an older age group, I feel, are essential for conducting such activities. Being in

good spirits is a responsibility. Not everyone comes just to exercise. Many need a lift that day, a chance to put aside their problems for just an hour, and that cannot happen if the instructor carries personal burdens into the classroom. I am not suggesting that we need to bounce through every class, operating on a supercharged energy level. But cheerfulness and enthusiasm are important to motivate our students and to make the program special and uplifting. Without question the leader sets the tone for the class hour. Those 60 minutes can drag or fly, depending on the atmosphere.

I recently watched a class during which the young instructor went through rather emotionless demonstrations, eyes downcast, addressing the floor rather than the students. No one was very comfortable, least of all the instructor. There was no bantering, no words of encouragement, no joking: This was serious business. No one needs this kind of exercise experience, regardless of age. Even if you are feeling blue, make sure your students are not affected. They come to feel better, not worse. It's easy to feel better as soon as the music and warm-up exercises start: faces light up, and smiles appear. From personal experience, I know that the saying "Sadness and activity are incompatible" is very true.

I have asked my students which instructor personality traits are important to them, and their comments are enlightening. They appreciate physical enthusiasm because it's catching and motivating. They want to feel that the instructor enjoys his or her work and enjoys being with them. They appreciate being treated as mature, intelligent adults. They love opportunities to laugh and let their hair down if the atmosphere set by the instructor is supportive. They prefer someone not too young: A certain amount of life experience, they feel, makes an instructor more sensitive to their needs and problems. A sense of humor is important. They appreciate someone with good listening and counseling skills and enough knowledge to deal with concerns and questions when they arise. Interest in one-to-one interaction is important, and a relationship of trust is high on the list. Most important is that the instructor be a caring, sensitive, and sincere person, comfortable with older people and concerned about each participant as an individual. The image of gym teachers as drill sergeants looms large in many people's minds; we can replace memories of whistle-blowing and rigid schoolyard drills with exercise time that is fun and meaningful.

be an educator

It's easy to be a performer before a class and impress students with graceful movements and physical ability. But it's much more important to educate them. It is not helpful to go through a series of motions without helping everyone understand why. Only through understanding can committed adherence to regular exercise develop. There is a great saying which I like to apply to exercise: "If you hear it, you forget; if you see it, you remember; but if you do it, you understand." And if the doing is reinforced by sufficient sharing of information, exercise will be understood and respected as what it really needs to be: an important factor in continued good health care. The information contained in this guide will serve as a basis for comfortably sharing important information about exercise, nutritional needs, and medical issues in the older years. It can easily be incorporated in your teaching in the form of short wellness lectures and will be appreciated by participants.

educating your students

I just spent some time rereading registration forms my students completed recently. One of my questions asks for a few comments about the program and what has been gained by participating. I am pleased to see that participants seem to truly appreciate my short talks, which are often accompanied by handouts. One person says, "The information-sharing and discussions always give me something to take home after class, something to think about, use, and pass on to my friends. I respond more to this kind of information than to reading articles because it is more personal."

I keep my talks brief and direct. Five minutes is usually enough time for sharing something new and interesting I have read, for offering useful nutritional or medical information, or for encouraging group discussion on a topic of interest. Handouts are always appreciated and can reinforce your short presentation.

Older participants are eager to listen, learn, and discuss. Chapters 11, 12, and 13 contain current and useful information you can share with your students. Additional reading will broaden your knowledge in these health-related areas and will help you prepare interesting presentations and handouts to reinforce what you have discussed.

teaching seniors: a challenge and reward

By deciding to work with seniors, we are accepting the challenge of being part of a pioneering effort. Exercise for the older generation is a relatively new venture, an area in which everyone proceeds with caution. Research will continue, but unless courageous and committed instructors are willing to set up programs

and act as catalysts and motivators, our seniors will not reap the benefits of healthful activity. It is exciting to be part of this movement to make exercise programs as available to our older generation as they are to younger ones. Replacing our apprehensions with common sense helps us meet this challenge. Exercise brings about improvement in all areas at all ages; no one is ever too old to benefit from physical movement. Seeing this improvement in our students' physical and mental well-being as a result of our teaching is a great reward and will keep us motivated. It's also nice to think that when we ourselves become seniors, there will be well-developed programs to help us stay active and healthy.

planning your classes

Even after 15 years of teaching, I cannot comfortably teach a class without adequate preparation. The longer I teach, the more I am confronted with the challenge of keeping my classes imaginative. It's easy to let ourselves get into a rut. Many instructors prefer to develop set routines that they "train" their students to remember: a certain set of warm-ups, predictable abdominal exercises, a never-changing set of stretches, and so on. This way, much preparation work is eliminated. If music resources are limited, even this tool, which can be a source of real exercise stimulation, becomes dull. Classes become predictable events, lacking in fun, surprises, and flexibility. To avoid this, we need to make a commitment to thorough and creative planning for each class we teach.

I have always been fascinated to observe how many participants in all my classes, and especially in the seniors' class, move to the beat of different drummers. Their coordination may not be great, or they may have little sense of rhythm when it comes to moving to music. Reaction time is not as fast in some as in others. Size, shape, and physical limitations create variables in movement patterns. To expect a group of individuals in various states of physical condition and health, especially at an older age, to perform like cheerleaders is unreasonable and purposeless. Learning routines is cumbersome and frustrating to most and only serves to point out those with coordination problems, making them feel clumsy and inept. It takes away opportunities for spontaneous movement and does not leave room for individual differences. It takes time to learn routines, and even if just two people don't catch on, the whole group is affected.

My first suggestion, for all these reasons, is to keep things simple and manageable. The purpose of exercise for seniors is to move all joints through their full range of motion, to improve muscle tone, strength, and flexibility, and to increase endurance. If we allow each person to move in his or her most comfortable way, the exercise benefits will be greatest. It is, of course, important to combine movement sequences that connect and are logical in their progression. In this sense, there is a need for choreography of a simple, sensible nature. Even a combination of very basic exercise movements can look very nice and make everyone feel graceful. In this guide, I have made exercise suggestions in groupings of connecting movements to help develop this basic concept of simple choreography.

As I plan my classes, I look at the exercise hour as a pie that I can divide into a number of segments with a certain amount of flexibility as to the size of each. There should be five segments: warm-up exercises, muscle strengthening and flexibility exercises, endurance activities, limbering and stretching, and cooling down and relaxation. This basic skeleton can be padded in a great variety of ways, drawing from the many suggestions contained in this guide and from your personal "arsenal" of exercises and creative ideas.

warm-up exercises

Warm-up exercises serve to slowly increase heart rate and blood circulation, warm muscles, limber and lubricate joints, and prepare the body for more demanding exercises and activities. In your planning, think of "shifting gears" as you would in your car: Don't race out of your driveway in third or fourth. The engine warms up in first gear, and you know by its sound when to shift. If you do it right, there will be no bumping or sputtering; transition from one gear to the next is smooth and easy. Common sense and warm-up exercises belong together. This important segment of the class does not make specific exercise demands. It simply prepares muscles, joints, and the cardiovascular system for the activities ahead. It's a "wake-up" time for the whole system and brings a glow to each face, a feeling of readiness to the body. It helps prevent injuries because warmed muscles are more efficient and flexible. Never skimp on this portion of your class; 5 to 10 minutes of preparation are not a waste of exercise time.

muscle strengthening and flexibility exercises

General muscle strengthening and joint range of motion exercises should be part of every fitness program. Popular aerobic programs often do not spend enough time with these important fitness components, resulting in unbalanced exercising. To attain and maintain a healthful level of overall fitness at every age, we have to place demands on major muscle groups and all joints, not just on the heart and lungs. All basic components of fitness are important, and with thorough preparation each area can be addressed in each class. Maintenance of strength and overall mobility is of great importance for staying independent and physically self-confident. Older people tend to lose this self-confidence as the years go by. The feeling "I can't do what I used to" prevails because the physical work that was part of the younger years has been replaced by a lifestyle of lazy leisure living. Disuse results in loss of strength and range of motion, but the ability to improve is there for everyone at every age. Restoring physical self-confidence is certainly possible and especially rewarding and encouraging in the older years. Old muscles respond like young ones: They weaken with too little demand and strengthen with use. This segment of the exercise hour can include a great variety of exercises and activities aimed at using the major muscle groups and all joints. My planning here becomes specific only in terms of balancing these exercises well. Here, special needs within the group can be addressed. The strength and range of motion participants develop during this part of each class are tools for living better and more independently.

Hands and arms, shoulders, upper back, and chest; abdominals, lower back, hip flexors, and buttocks; thighs, calves, and feet—each of these should be exercised by the end of class. Fingers, wrists, shoulder joints, hip joints, knees, and ankles need range of motion exercises. I used to make a checklist for myself early in my teaching, and as I prepared a class, I would check off these different areas to have good exercise balance in each hour.

Stationary exercises for muscle strengthening tend to be dull and uninspiring, and this is where variety and creativity make the difference. There is no one specific exercise that is best for strengthening a certain muscle group: As long as muscles contract, strengthening takes place. Again, draw from the many suggestions in this guide and your own exercise reservoir to meet the goals for this portion of your class.

endurance activities

Endurance activities are popularly called aerobics. These activities make demands on the cardiorespiratory system—the heart and lungs. The heart is a muscle and responds to exercise much like other muscles, and appropriate activities can bring great improvements in its strength and efficiency. All daily tasks become easier because blood is pumped more efficiently to all tissues. Guidelines for safe cardiorespiratory exercise are contained in the medical chapter of this manual.

Everyone in my classes enjoys this portion of the exercise hour best. It's an "up" time, a time for having fun as a group, for generating energy and putting pep into everyone's steps. I make great efforts to introduce a variety of activities during this segment so that there is always something new to look forward to. Exposure to different kinds of movement—elements of square dance, folk dance, African dance, and Scottish dance, for example—can help generate new ideas, and that's how the spark stays in our programs.

As I plan for the next day's class, I consider a number of things. Weather and temperature, for example, significantly influence energy levels. Here in the Connecticut Valley, humidity is very high for a number of months and oxygen content low. Even at a fairly low level of exertion, heart rates go up quickly and breathing becomes difficult. I alternate activities that require a little more effort with less demanding work. To accommodate these variables, jogging can turn into comfortable "slogging," and a light run into a brisk walk. But I keep everyone up and moving for at least 20 minutes, slowing down to a walking pace toward the end so that heart rates begin to go down.

limbering, stretching, and cooling down

Limbering, stretching, and cooling down should take about 10 minutes, and again there are no limits as to how you can fill this segment of the class hour. Working with partners is a sociable, fun way to stretch and cool down. We often use hand equipment for effective stretching, bending, and twisting. The purpose of whatever you choose to do during this time is to bring heart rate and breathing back to normal after the demands of endurance work, to bring body temperature down, and to stretch tight muscle groups.

The last 5 minutes are reserved for "going limp," for letting muscles go slack, for consciously experiencing that good feeling of pleasant tiredness after an hour's exercise. I like to bring everyone together for these last few minutes and choose slow, relaxing music we can hum or sing along with. There is a good feeling of togetherness after having shared the hour, and everyone can leave feeling well exercised and relaxed. We often stay in our circle for another few minutes to share some interesting news or to talk about what was most enjoyable during the hour. Realizing that everyone is feeling well at the end of a class continues to be a source of great joy for me, reinforcing the value of thoughtful planning.

sequence and progression of exercises and activities

Within each segment of the exercise hour, there needs to be a logical sequence of progression. The lesson outlines provided in Appendix A progress from one set of exercises to the next. Again, the best suggestion I can make is to "shift gears," start easily, progress slowly, and not make things too demanding. Common sense in progression should continue to guide you as the weeks go by. Improved strength and endurance are the result of *regular, moderate* exercise, and each class hour adds one more building block to what may initially have been a shaky foundation. A low level of fitness needs an initial prescription of low-level activity. It doesn't take much to overload unused muscles, stiff joints, and a weak cardiorespiratory system. Increases in small increments help the body adapt and become ready for more demanding work.

For improvements to take place, exercise has to impose reasonable demands. The body adapts to the imposed load by becoming stronger, and the load can then be increased. The amount of improvement is directly related to how often, how long, and how hard a person exercises. This is as true for the senior participant as it is for the professional athlete. Work load and fitness levels obviously cannot compare, but the physiological process is the same. "Train, don't strain!" is important advice for all exercisers. Nothing is gained by rushing head-on into a fitness program. Sensibly progressing over a number of months assures safe participation with healthful results. It prevents people from becoming exercise dropouts due to feeling unsuccessful, frustrated, exhausted, sore, or being injured. Because you may not know what your students' level of physical condition is as you begin your program, it's best to *start easy and progress slowly*, introducing exercise as positively and enjoyably as possible. If the first few classes lay a positive foundation by having everyone feel capable and successful, your students will be hooked and will look forward to coming back.

HAVING FUN is spelled in giant letters as I plan my classes. When I ask the seniors with whom I work what they enjoy most about our program, the chorus of "It's so much fun!" convinces me that dreaming up new and different ways of having fun is worth the trouble. The endurance segment of the class provides the best opportunity for playing and feeling like kids—something the world out there doesn't really approve of when you are 70 or 80. "Act your age" is what is expected, and skipping down supermarket aisles is not a publicly accepted option.

What I see my older students discover is that there is a part of their personalities that remained youthful—spontaneous, fun-loving, playful, and silly. To be in an environment supportive of all those things again, of skipping along without being judged odd, of "playing" in a group of people who thoroughly enjoy each other can shed years in a flash. Here I truly see exercise being the proverbial fountain of youth: It's there for the taking, and it works. It's the best pep pill and turns even a reclusive person into a cheerful participant. "There is something important I have learned in this class: to laugh!" one woman not usually given to expressing emotions said to me recently. In our class she can't resist being part of that light, happy atmosphere, and her initial apprehension has been replaced with sincere enjoyment.

music for moving in rhythm

Music can make or break a fitness class. If well chosen, it sets the perfect mood for your planned activities. The right music can mean the difference between enthusiastic participation or half-hearted attempts at making it through the hour. It inspires the body to move more correctly and easily, helps those with poor coordination by providing a dependable beat, and makes exercise more than a physical workout. Well-selected music makes the hour emotionally uplifting and affects both body and mind positively, a combination to strive for in our teaching.

Music selection is relatively easy if you teach younger classes. Current pop, rock, jazz, and country music hits are popular and enthusiastically received for high-energy aerobic workouts. But to appeal to our older students, we have to search in the music archives of the past in addition to being very selective with more current music. It's a challenge to find the right variety of music to appeal to this generation and to stay away from what for many is a nerve-wracking noise experience. Many of my older students react very negatively to certain instrumentation and sound levels. Poorly selected music can be a source of stress and can inhibit motivation and spontaneous, joyful participation.

Music search and selection can be a very time-consuming (and, unfortunately, expensive) part of our work. But the time and energy spent on making good selections is invaluable. No matter how accomplished and well prepared the instructor may be in all other areas, poor musical selections can ruin a well-planned class in short order by frustrating participants and making potentially high spirits fall. Music has to inspire participation instantly. It has to keep everyone going for the class hour, inspire the urge to move and snap fingers, and provide a good variety of rhythms to make all movements feel right. It's like dancing: You can't dance the rhumba to a waltz beat without getting confused and ill-tempered, feeling like a klutz, and stepping on your partner's feet. Think about and listen carefully to each piece of music you take into the classroom to make sure it complements the exercises and movements you have planned. Select music your students will enjoy and appreciate; ask for suggestions and feedback instead of relying only on personal taste. It's always good to keep foremost in mind that we teach to stimulate our students, not to satisfy our own tastes.

If you know that your musical sense is poor, that you cannot easily distinguish good rhythms from bad and have little natural ability for working with music, try to find someone who can help you. It's too important to leave it to chance. Don't make it easy by just tuning in to your favorite radio station to have background music. Your students depend on good selections and basic choreography to enjoy the class hour and get the most from it.

I feel most organized and well prepared by making tapes of music, selecting and combining appropriate pieces for the lesson I have planned. Everyone loves popular renditions of familiar classical pieces. Broadway music, folk and country, contra dance, and pretty instrumental pieces can be combined into a colorful potpourri that contains something for every taste. If budget or personal music selection are limited, try to borrow records from friends or class members. Your local library's music section is another resource worth exploring. I have even found our local radio station willing to lend me some of their older records that were stored away and collecting dust. I have made music suggestions in Appendix B, and you may find many of these records as "oldies but goodies" at tag sales or at record stores that sell used, reasonably priced records.

Making tapes is a lot of work, but once planning and taping is completed, you can add this new program to your permanent library of taped lessons. I have built up a selection of about 20 taped programs for my seniors classes, and a work sheet to go with each, outlining the exercises and activities appropriate for the music. When I get tired of certain music selections, I can tape over these, replacing them with new and more enjoyable pieces. I still make a completely new tape occasionally but basically have an adequate music library to draw from and add variety by replacing some selections regularly and changing the exercises. I make special tapes for special occasions like Christmas when we go through our paces while singing "Jingle Bells" and other favorites. These 45-minute tapes provide enough music for a one-hour class. Taping helps you to carefully plan a sequence and progression of exercises while keeping flexibility in your program. It's much like preparing notes for a lecture: It's all there as an outline, giving you a basic skeleton with which to work but leaving you with enough flexibility for changes each time you use this skeleton.

I find it very important to work with the music at home before taking it into the classroom. A beat that sounds right for walking may turn out to be just a little too slow or too fast when you walk along with it for a minute. A peppy beat apparently perfect for warm-up exercises may actually leave you breathless when you try it out at home. A slow, melancholy piece can make you feel low and draggy after several minutes of listening, rather than having a positive, relaxing effect. If a selection is too long, it can become boring and repetitious, and I rarely record anything that's longer than 2-1/2 to 3 minutes. Listen to the lyrics and decide whether there's a positive message—woeful country lyrics, for example, are not very uplifting. To please a variety of tastes, try to combine a variety of musical styles. There is so much to choose from.

Music can be a prime motivator and inspire you to think of new things to do. Keep listening to radio stations with a "conservative" listener approach, and simply call the station for music titles if they are not announced. Stay open-minded instead of relying only on your personal music preferences. I don't particularly love listening to country music at home but find it refreshing and fun in my teaching. If classical music is your preference, recognize that most of it was not composed for sit-ups or leg kicks. Most classical music does not provide a consistent beat or rhythm to exercise to, but many favorite pieces have been brought up-to-date with a good beat, and I have listed some in my music suggestions. Take advantage of the wonderful options a variety of music can add to your teaching and accept the challenge to become an expert in selecting just the right music for "Senior Harmony" in your classes.

The rewards of spending time and energy on overall planning are great. If we follow common sense, consider special needs in our group, carefully look at sequence and progression, make FUN the main ingredient, and use music our students enjoy and appreciate, it will be easy to teach a successful program.

know your students

People in my classes marvel at my ability to remember names. A variety of things help. Everyone completes a registration form giving information that is specific and personal. I have a conversation with each new class member to help me remember something special about him or her. I will remember that Mary shares my love for perennial gardening, that Steve has a rowing machine at home that he uses daily, that Ann loves to wear purple. Fortunately, most classes start small with a reasonable number of names to remember. Beyond that, I only have to remember one or two names at a time as new people join. I also keep a sign-in sheet on my work table, and as people arrive, they check in. This is always a good time for short one-to-one exchanges. After a number of weeks, I have little reason or excuse not to remember their names. It's nice to feel individual in a group, to know that the instructor cares enough to remember our names and something about us, to hear "Hi, Mary!" instead of an impersonal hello. I also am never embarrassed to ask if I draw a mental blank. If remembering names is not your specialty, consider having everyone wear nametags for the first few classes. It helps all participants in getting to know each other by name.

For overall information about each person, I ask for completion of a registration form. I am most concerned about health history and present health status, medication, physical limitations, name of physician, and so forth. If anything is unclear, I spend enough time with the person to be more fully informed. When necessary, I contact the physician to be assured that he or she supports the patient's participation in our exercise program. I like to know about my students' exercise and self-care attitudes and habits, what they hope to gain from participation in the program, which improvements they feel they need, and so on. Basically, I try to find out as much as possible without intruding. This personal information gives me a better basis for developing a relationship with individuals.

The most meaningful way of getting to know your students, of course, is through one-to-one interaction. Opportunities for personal conversations can be created by being in the classroom before your students arrive and by puttering around for a while at the end of the class. If people know that you are there early, those in need of talking will appear, and the stragglers who stay after class probably are staying for a reason. Again, it's up to us to be sensitive and aware, to take opportunities offered, and to draw people into conversation.

Several years ago, I bought a good upright scale. Once a week I offer to weigh those who are interested. Obviously, no one needs my help; but here is another opportunity for brief but regular one-to-one contacts, and exchanging even a few sentences helps me stay aware of good happenings, problems and pains, exciting travel plans, and, of course, weight gain. But the scale readout doesn't really seem very important to anyone, even though many will lament if the indicator climbs a little higher than the previous week. I know it's the personal interaction that makes our scales a very popular item.

There is one tool that, in my experience, is most powerful and special in drawing individuals into a comfortable relationship: physical touching. I have found that older persons are much more open to physical touching than those of my own age, perhaps because so many live alone. In our classrooms we can create the right atmosphere for some comfortable physical interaction. Bumper stickers encourage us to hug our dogs, cats, nurses, and plumbers. Let's add senior citizens to the list—they need it most.

Finally, a most important way to get to know our students is by developing good listening skills. It's tempting to be a talker when you are a teacher: After all, people are there for instruction and direction. But you don't learn much about others by talking. To learn, you have to listen.

Just as the need for touching is there, the need to be listened to and, if possible, to be given some simple advice is very strong, especially in people who live alone. A caring, trusting relationship between you and your students will make this interaction possible. These situations, especially regarding medical questions and personal counseling, concerned me until I spoke to friends in the medical profession. They assured me that given my concern for and relationship with participants, I should be in a good position to advise, and, as a result, I now feel more comfortable in that role. I try to guide the conversation in such a way that people answer their own questions, something I learned from getting my children through their teenage years. If I cannot comfortably answer a question immediately, I promise to find out. For more complicated situations, I will direct the person to professional help. If we are guided by common sense and recognize our personal limitations for advising, we can often help someone who needs a listening ear and a caring heart.

continuing self-education

At this time, I am not aware of a specific educational process that prepares fitness instructors for working with seniors. But as this segment of our population continues to grow, the need for appropriately prepared educators will become obvious. For now, those of us interested in this work have to patch together our own education. We can do good work if we make every effort to be as knowledgeable as is presently possible about issues relating to older persons' health and exercise needs. Articles on health, exercise, diet, and aging appear in every popular magazine now, and it's often difficult to judge whether these materials are dependably accurate. It's hard to distinguish the scientifically based information from the merely fashionable unless we have a solid reading foundation. Books and other materials I have listed in Appendix C are current, come from respected sources, and give scientifically accurate information as it now exists. Such resource material should be on every instructor's bookshelf to ensure basic, accurate knowledge in the areas of exercise, nutrition, wellness, and aging. New publications will continue to appear, helping all of us to stay current and informed.

I have been fortunate to live in an academic community with opportunities to take courses that help me in my work. If there is a university or college near you, inform yourself about course offerings that would broaden your knowledge. Exercise physiology, nutrition, anthropology, gerontology, psychology—all these subject areas are of importance and interest when working with older people. The more you know, the better your program will be and the more secure you will feel relating to and advising your older students.

instructor network

As is true in all types of work, sharing knowledge, experiences, and problem situations with colleagues is very helpful. It's something I have missed greatly in my work with seniors. Very few programs exist in our geographic area, and those who teach seem to be very isolated, not necessarily aware of each other's existence. I hope that regional networks for instructors will be established in the future so that we can meet with others, learn from them, share what we know, and support each other. It's hard to rely just on one's own resources year after year and stay enthusiastic. I do attend general fitness leadership workshops when possible, but not many are offered, and they rarely include special sessions on work with seniors. You may want to establish your own instructor network if there are other programs in your general area or organize occasional informal workshops for supporting each other and to renew enthusiasm for your work.

First aid and CPR courses, fortunately, are offered everywhere and give you the knowledge and confidence to deal with a possible problem situation. I have been extremely fortunate in my many years of teaching. With just a few dizzy spells, an occasional fall without injury, a sprained ankle, or a pulled muscle, I have not had much practice in applying my first aid and CPR skills. But my medical friends always remind me that the law of averages will have to catch up with me. As I keep my certifications up-to-date and my wits about me throughout every class, I hope for another decade of teaching without major problems.

resources in your community

Whether you are volunteering your time and energy or are hired to teach a program in your community, there will be an organization behind you to help in a variety of ways. Most commonly, activities for seniors are sponsored by YMCAs, local councils on aging, Jewish community centers, or recreation departments. I have a close working relationship with our council on aging. The program director secured our present space, a large church hall, free of charge by meeting with church board members. A monthly newsletter mailed to all seniors includes information about our program and special announcements I want to make. Concerns I may have had about lawsuits and insurance issues are eliminated because I am covered by a general town policy. Occasional workshop fees or material costs are covered by squeezing an always tight senior center budget. These issues of space, insurance, publicity, and expense are important in setting up a new program and for being supported and feeling appreciated, especially as a volunteer. Senior center personnel are important resource persons. They are familiar with a range of professional services in the community and often have a social worker on their staff who is available for counseling or can give information and suggestions when needed. I find it very helpful at times to brainstorm with someone at the senior center if one of my students is going through a difficult time and needs help and support. Staff members know most of the participants in my

program and may have insights I am lacking. Even though I do not teach in the senior center building, my visits are regular and my contacts with staff persons always helpful.

Being informed about the medical professionals in the community has been very important. I have made it a point to establish contact with those specialists older persons would be most likely to consult. I have interviewed many for a health column I write, and this has given me a special opportunity to make personal contacts and to introduce myself and my work. I then feel comfortable making a phone call if I need a medical opinion or if someone needs to be directed to the appropriate source of help.

I try to arrange for occasional lectures by local professionals. A young podiatrist in the community comes in to offer advice on common foot problems. His yearly presentations are informative and helpful. A local internist with a busy practice agreed to a presentation on doctor-patient relationships. A nutrition professor shared important information on dietary needs in aging, and a massage therapist instructed us in simple tension-releasing partner massage techniques. Understandably, it is not easy to find physicians who are available for daytime lectures, and we can't have the variety of medical information-sharing I would like. Professionals in the community might be more willing to make their contributions to educating seniors if evening lectures could be arranged.

Even if it is not possible to meet members of your local medical community in person, you can keep your ears open and find out some basic information. It is important to know who is good with older patients, who has an open-file approach and educates patients, who is supportive of activity at an older age, and who is strongly preventively oriented. The best we can do is to be a source of basic information and to steer people in the right direction if they come to us with questions.

the classroom challenge

Not everyone I see in my classes comes without initial reluctance and apprehension. Many have never before participated in a fitness program, and the word *exercise* is not part of their vocabulary as it is for younger people. Hard physical work in earlier life makes many feel that they deserve rest rather than exertion at this stage in their lives. My mother was a good example. She raised five children and enough chickens, rabbits, and vegetables to feed us year around. She worked hard from morning to night without push-button conveniences. There was no need for additional exercise in her life, and encouraging her to join a fitness program in her later years would have taken some doing. She did, however, watch my classes with great interest during her visits from Germany and recognized that her heart condition and circulatory problems would benefit from more activity. Instinctively, everyone seems to know that exercise is important for better health at every stage of life.

Those who are inclined to take it easy can always find a long list of reasons for not activating themselves. Many people are literally dragged to class by friends who have become exercise converts. These more active folks have often nagged their sedentary friends for months, elaborating on how much fun their class is, how much better they feel, and how important it has become to build this regular exercise into each week. Sometimes the nagging is successful, resistance buckles, and a potential new participant appears—"just to watch." Then I must rise to the challenge and present our program in the most positive way in order to draw this reluctant bystander into our midst.

class atmosphere

This situation arises with regularity, and it is the classroom atmosphere that will affect the newcomer's decision to join us or not. A comfortable atmosphere doesn't just happen when you bring a group of people together; it has to be created. Everyone has the same hopes for a new situation: to feel welcome and comfortable. It's our responsibility to create the right atmosphere, to be aware of how much control we have over setting the tone.

If the instructor is at ease before the group, everyone else can relax. Cheerfulness, a light touch with people, and a sense of humor contribute greatly to the comfort level in the classroom. From personal experience I know that physical education teachers can be forceful, intimidating, and often cutting in their humor, making gym class a difficult experience for many. Good teachers do not need to resort to these negative tools, and in working with older adults, such approaches are totally inappropriate. A sense of humor is a wonderful tool to help everyone feel at ease—if it's in good taste and respectful of the group. We want our students to enjoy the class, to have fun and share laughter instead of experiencing exercise as a serious event.

I prefer a chatty atmosphere in all my classes and begin to worry when silence hangs over the room. My immediate assumption is that I am on the wrong track, which is usually true. Flexibility in planning then pays off because I am prepared to change direction in midstream to improve the atmosphere. Instead of persisting with the lesson plan, I change to activities that, from experience, I am sure everyone enjoys more. Group or partner activities foster the return to socialization and encourage chatty conversations. Momentary discomforts can be removed by giving everyone a chance for interaction or by asking for suggestions. It's easy to say, "I have a feeling that you are not having a lot of fun this morning. What would you like to do instead to have a better time?" When students have no inhibitions about speaking up, the lesson then takes a positive turn.

These practical considerations affect atmosphere, but the real groundwork for a successful program is laid by our approach to our students. Respect for the older generation seems to have been lost in the shuffle of fast living. There's not enough time to get to know our elders, listen to them, and appreciate them. Stories of "the olden days" are a bore to many young people. There seems little interest in advice from elders or in learning from their lifelong experiences. All of us who work with older people have great opportunities to help make changes in these attitudes, and treating each individual with sincere respect is a key ingredient. We are fortunate and privileged to have limitless opportunities for growing and learning through these contacts, for being positively influenced in how we approach our own aging, and for forming very genuine relationships. "When we talk about old age, each of us is talking about his or her own future," says Dr. Robert Butler in his book *Why Survive? Being Old In America*. His reminder should stay with us at all times as we work with seniors.

If respect is part of a relationship, it's easy to trust. My students know that I respect their ability, limitations, good decision-making skills, maturity, and intelligence. In turn, they will trust me completely to safely guide them through each class. This trust has enabled me to explore and experiment, knowing that students will react and critique honestly and openly. They know that their well-being is my guide in teaching, that I would not suggest activities that are unsafe, purposeless, or foolish. This trust, in addition to being based on respect, is also greatly inspired by an overall feeling of caring. They know that I do this work because it comes from the heart, because I feel privileged working with them, and because I sincerely appreciate the resulting relationships. What happens in our classroom is positive human interaction: We set and meet challenges in an atmosphere of friendship and develop group cohesiveness by respecting, liking, and trusting each other. I am part of the group, not apart from it, always remembering that "it's nice to be important, but more important to be nice."

motivating your students

In evaluating the many tools that seem important to do this work well, one great challenge is to find ways of motivating all students to test their physical abilities and to continue attending week after week. It helps to look at what motivates us personally when we become involved in new endeavors. Experiences should be stimulating and challenging, for the mind as well as the body. If this new venture is in a classroom setting, encouragement from the instructor like an occasional pat on the back and a good progress report is appreciated. Feeling successful is a great motivator. All these criteria can be met in our fitness classes, assuring adherence for long enough to experience noticeable changes. Once we have helped participants over the initial hurdles every beginning exerciser faces, the improved physical and mental well-being becomes self-generated motivation for continued participation. I love hearing the general lamenting as we end our last class in June: "We are going to fall apart over the summer! It will feel terrible not to exercise regularly! We'll miss seeing everyone! We are going to get fat and flabby!" These are strong expressions of positive "exercise addiction." Rather than *hoping* to see everyone again in September, I can be confident that I *will*. My phone will start to ring in late August: "Just want to make sure we are starting next week—I don't want to miss our first class!" If everyone looks forward to getting back to a pattern of living that includes this structured regular exercise, we can be sure of having done our work well.

The one tremendous advantage we have in teaching adults is that everyone is there as a result of personal choice. By joining, they have expressed the desire to be there, to make improvements in their general lifestyle and self-care. I came to fully appreciate this fact when volunteering at our local high school for a semester. The general attitude was one of having no choice—this class was just another part of a long school day to get through. I never quite lost the feeling that my presence was inflicted on the students. I often had to do physical and mental somersaults to get a spark of enthusiasm ignited, something I rarely experience in my adult classes. I had to push hard to make everyone move and often felt quite unsuccessful and not very appreciated. In contrast, working with older, enthusiastic, and appreciative participants is a joy!

I encourage and receive input and feedback to help me set the right pace for our class. One of my students recently called me a "baby senior citizen," a nice term for a middle-aged instructor! I am 20 to 30 years younger than most of my senior students and in good

physical condition. I cannot rely on my own physical responses to the exercise demands to understand what my older students are experiencing but must rely on their input. The classroom atmosphere makes open communication between us very comfortable. They tell me when they are beginning to run out of steam and are ready for something less demanding. I regularly "check in" with the class by asking if we are working too hard, not hard enough, or if the pace feels just right. There is honest reaction to activities they don't enjoy very much, and the simple solution is to eliminate those. I am as observant as I can be, but I urge everyone to take the responsibility to help and guide me instead of confronting me with a general collapse because I was not perceptive enough. And reminders come: They would like to spend more time with relaxation exercises at the end, I haven't brought in some of their favorite music for a while, the music was too loud, our experimenting with ankle weights didn't appeal to the majority. This feedback has helped me eliminate many exercises, replacing them with more appropriate ones. Basically, we have experimented together and have cooperatively developed a sensible, safe, and enjoyable program.

right place, right time

My work takes me from one exercise space to another in the course of a week. My first gym was located in an abandoned school building with a leaking roof and poor heat. We had buckets set up in strategic places to catch the water when it rained and wore mittens and sweaters in winter. I have been in basement church halls with dirty floors, obstructive pillars, and no windows. We have exercised in club halls where wedding parties left floors coated with spilled food and drinks, and in spaces without heat control or ventilation. Of the many factors that affect a fitness program, physical environment is a very powerful one. I no longer agree to teach in spaces that deflate my high spirits as soon as I walk through the door.

I realize that finding the perfect place can be a tremendous hurdle and that we often have to settle for less to get a program started. But keeping some basic considerations in mind is important. First, the room needs to be large enough to allow everyone to move about freely. Even if the number of participants is fairly small in the beginning, a certain amount of space is absolutely necessary for endurance activities. It's hard to keep moving along if you run into a wall after every few steps, and walking or running in small circles is a dizzying experience and certainly neither fun nor safe. A small space imposes great limitations on activity choices and restricts freedom of movement. It also immediately limits the number of participants, and interested newcomers have to be turned away.

Safety is next on the list. If there are stairs to the building or hall, are they in good repair? Are they cleared of snow and ice before class begins? Is the floor in good condition, or are there loose or missing tiles? Is it sticky, or too slick with wax and polish? Are there obstacles someone could trip over? How is the lighting? These are things to investigate carefully.

Then, get a feeling for the atmosphere in this space. Does a lack of windows make it stuffy, dark, and depressing? Or is the sun shining in and a breeze blowing through open windows, making everything bright and cheerful? Is there a thermostat you can control? Despite rising heat costs, many public spaces are still very overheated, which is unhealthy and energy-robbing during exercise. (Whenever I look for new space, our low heat demands are a real selling point. I always keep the thermostat at around 55°, a comfortable temperature for everyone during exercise.)

I also take a close look at the cleanliness of the floor. I find carpeted halls unappealing and unhygienic for floor exercises and less safe for endurance activities. Always make friends with custodians. Their willingness to keep floors sparkling clean is so important, especially if other activities have taken place before your class. No other group has the same need for well-washed floors because they don't sit or lie down on them. There is nothing worse than finding your nose in food or bubble gum.

Space location, too, is important to consider. If at all possible, try to find a centrally located hall with adequate parking space and easy access to the building. Should community space be needed, it is most helpful to have the organization make this request for you. Boards of churches or clubs are more likely to respond positively to a request made by the Council on Aging than by an individual because of insurance issues and because of their willingness to help nonprofit causes. But be involved in looking at available spaces: You will have to teach there so you should feel safe and comfortable with the arrangement. If at all possible, find a hall with folding chairs. Chairs are great for a wide variety of exercises, and you will use them often.

The last question is meeting time: when, how often, and for how long? I have found that holding a 1-hour class twice a week works out best. Some, because of other involvements, cannot come both days. But the majority do, and I strongly encourage this commitment. A Monday/Thursday or Tuesday/Friday schedule works well. If a full hour's exercise seems too much, take short exercise breaks for health-related information sharing and group discussion.

3
basic fitness components and exercise equipment

Good overall fitness has a number of components, and with the current national emphasis on endurance activities, it is easy to forget the importance of keeping a healthy balance in our exercise programs. A runner faithfully committed to his or her daily mileage will not be strong and flexible unless he or she specifically works at it. The weight lifter with strong, well-defined muscles may not be able to run around the block. Those adhering to a daily routine of push-ups and sit-ups can have more body fat than is healthy. Exercises and activities need to be balanced to build a good foundation for overall fitness, and this foundation can still be developed or improved at an older age. What we need to keep in mind, however, is that exercise intensity and goals for an older population are different from those of young or middle-aged persons, so it is not possible to apply a general formula.

cardiorespiratory fitness

Cardiorespiratory fitness, or aerobic fitness, has been established as the foundation of overall well-being. All activities that place adequate demands on heart and lungs have far-reaching benefits. Extensive research suggests reduced risk of heart disease if such conditioning is developed and maintained throughout adult life. Circulation and breathing are greatly improved and resting heart rate is lowered, indicating that the heart pumps blood more efficiently. Food is metabolized more efficiently, which aids in controlling body weight. Bones, ligaments, and tendons are strengthened through weight-bearing activities, making the exerciser less susceptible to fractures, sprains, and joint injury. Endurance activities put pep into our step, increase energy and vigor, and help work off stress and tension. Heart and lung fitness give us increased capacity for participating in life and for meeting a variety of demands with energy left over for leisure activities. We sleep better and feel better throughout the day. "Running out of steam" is a rare experience for the person in good cardiorespiratory condition.

Aerobic exercise is prescribed by physicians and psychiatrists to remedy a range of ills, including depression and the need for tranquilizers. The person feels in charge, is more productive, and experiences increased self-esteem. Exercise, in general, is a positive substitute for smoking, drinking, or overeating, and aerobic activities help greatly in changing these poor health habits. But can aerobic fitness be achieved in the later years? We see young people jogging, playing tennis or racquetball, speeding along on racing bikes, and joining aerobic dance programs everywhere to develop long-term cardiovascular health. At 70, not many are likely to participate in such activities, and it is understandable that the older generation does not feel included in the aerobic fitness movement. Those who have led a rather sedentary retirement life will feel that they are beyond the demands of aerobic exercising, and that taking it easy and preserving energy is the safer way to live.

Good fitness programs for seniors can help remove these apprehensions and open doors to a healthier, more energetic way of life. Older participants can experience the physical and mental benefits of safe and appropriate endurance activities that are tailored to their needs and abilities. Improvements come with regular participation, and attitudes change if we present sensible programs and set reachable goals. Starting easily, building up slowly, and not exceeding the age-related guidelines established for endurance exercise is the approach to take at any age.

frequency, intensity, and duration

The right frequency, intensity, duration, and kind of exercise for older participants clearly depends on the individual. When determining exercise intensity, researchers divide the older population into three basic groups:

1. The "old old" are individuals who are in need of nursing home care and support and are 75 years or older.

2. The "young old" are persons who still live in their own homes in the community and are between 60 and 75 years old.
3. The "athletic old" are the small percentage of older individuals who have maintained a high degree of physical fitness and still participate in sports activities.

These tremendous ranges in health, physical condition, and ability make clear that exercise prescription for the older adult has to contain a great deal of flexibility and individual consideration; therefore, we should not expect uniform participation in our programs. The wide range of physical abilities makes self-monitoring important, and we must educate our older students in this process so that their participation is safe and health-promoting.

perceived exertion

Discussing the importance of *perceived exertion*, the awareness of personal physical response to exercise demands, is a priority. If the exercise or activity is perceived as being too difficult, it probably is, and slowing down or resting for a while is a logical, healthy reaction. "Listen to your body!" is important advice. We should always remind participants to rely on physical signals and use good judgment in response. Each individual is the best judge for evaluating degree of effort by how it feels. This, in addition to knowing how to take an exercise pulse, gives each person a good basis for personal decision making in a group setting.

When discussing this important issue, I strongly encourage everyone to deal with our class activities no differently than they would with physical work at home. After a certain amount of yard or housework, there is a natural need and desire to stop and rest. If the work is too demanding and causes muscular fatigue, a very elevated heart rate, or labored breathing, the normal reaction is to put aside this particular chore. There should be no pressure in our classrooms to cause decision making to be any less sensible. Eliminating all pressures to perform or compete and not setting specific expectations are important considerations. I have found my students to be very sensible, aware of individual limitations, and protective of their well-being. Knowing that I strongly support their nonparticipation and completely trust their decision making, everyone feels free to do as much or as little as feels right on any given day. This trust in their good judgment has given me the confidence to encourage regular participation in endurance activities.

exercise prescription

In 1975, the American College of Sports Medicine established some basic guidelines for safe, beneficial aerobic exercise participation for seniors. Ideally, there should be 30 minutes of aerobic activity three to five times per week, and this could be walking, swimming, riding an exercise bike, or participating in an organized fitness program. Exercise heart rate is recommended to be at about 60% of maximum for the average, poorly conditioned older person.

A person's maximum heart rate shows a progressive decline from the age of about 25 years. The widely used formula of establishing an individual's maximum heart rate per minute is 220 − age in years. This means that at age 70, this maximum would be around 150 beats, compared to 180 at age 40. Exercising at 60% of this maximum would translate into an exercise heart rate of around 90 beats per minute. For many healthy, relatively fit older participants used to regular physical activity, house and yard work, or brisk walking, this may be quite low. The general American Heart Association guidelines suggest an exercise heart rate of 70 to 85% of the individual's maximum. This translates into 105 to 130 beats per minute for the 70-year-old. Keeping heart rate at the lower end of this range is probably advisable for those in poor physical condition, while those who are active, healthy, and fit may comfortably participate at the higher rate. Again, individual health status, level of physical condition, and perceived exertion need to guide the participant.

taking an exercise pulse

Because heart rate during exercise is a direct indicator of exercise intensity, it is important that all participants learn how to take their pulse, confidently and accurately. Participants must understand that this tool for occasional self-monitoring is important to avoid overexertion and consequent feelings of unwellness or exhaustion.

The beginning exerciser, no matter what the age, tends to have poor body awareness and little knowledge of physiology. Older participants in a structured fitness program with a knowledgeable leader can overcome this initial handicap if adequate education takes place in the classroom. Many older participants also have to overcome the additional handicap of the fear that exercise can cause problems. Depending on the instructor's approach in monitoring heart rate, this fear can either be intensified or alleviated.

Most aerobic conditioning programs take heart rate monitoring very seriously. In organized classes, participants are asked to stop their activity frequently for a 10-second pulse check. I do not agree with this approach for seniors even though general exercise guidelines make this recommendation. Not adhering to this advice has not caused any of my participants to suffer ill effects. I am not implying that this method of staying

in touch with exercise exertion is not important or that I disagree with the established guidelines. They are of great value to the middle-aged person who is concerned about the possible prevention of heart disease and wants to work at developing long-term aerobic fitness. In addition to keeping exercise intensity at a safe level, heart-rate monitoring can be a great motivator for the person beginning a program of aerobic activity. However, our older students' purpose and goals in exercise participation are of a different nature, and this is important to keep in mind. They should not be asked to push themselves to a certain pulse rate, nor should they feel that exercise will not benefit them unless they meet the recommended ''target zone'' pulse.

All movement is beneficial, and every hour of exercise adds to increasing the individual's present level of fitness, no matter what the heart rate. Insistence on constant monitoring results in presenting exercise to our older students as dangerous business to be approached with great caution. Common sense tells us that far greater problems arise from the lack of activity. Anything we can do to encourage older persons into regular, sensible activity will have health-promoting results, and we can help to eliminate existing apprehensions by educating those with whom we work.

Educating means encouraging self-responsibility. I do my best to provide information, to teach skills, and to encourage self-monitoring so that relying on perceived exertion becomes a clear guide in everyone's participation. I trust participants to respond to what they experience physically and to make good decisions on that basis. For some individuals this may mean taking their pulse occasionally while activity is increased. For most, perceived exertion becomes a secure guide throughout the hour. On the whole, I am not comfortable with the insistence on group pulse taking and feel that it leaves a fearful atmosphere in the classroom. My discussions with physicians have supported these feelings, and I know that my students are very comfortable with this approach.

Obviously, each instructor has to approach this issue in a manner which feels right or which is necessary due to the sponsoring organization's policy, and I am only sharing my personal feelings. I do make sure that a clock with a second hand is in the classroom and that each new participant receives information providing a basic understanding of cardiovascular exercise and recommended guidelines. On hot and humid days, I remind everyone to take his or her pulse because the weather imposes greater stress on the cardiovascular system. On the whole, I trust each individual to take charge, just as they would in doing physical work, spending an evening square dancing, or going out for a long walk—normal activities for which no one would urge heart rate monitoring but which are just as demanding as this hour of organized activity.

I often feel that individuals are encouraged to relinquish too much responsibility and become increasingly less responsible for themselves, out of touch with who they are and what they feel. Most older persons would not consider exercising at a pace or level of exertion that could be injurious to their well-being. We younger, much less sensible folks insist on pushing ourselves to the limit, running races and marathons, doing 200 sit-ups in a row, and pumping iron to the point of exhaustion. I have great trust in the older generation's more cautious approach to exercise participation and less concern about their overdoing, being injured, or having heart attacks. It is the middle-aged males, frantically trying to turn back the clock or make up for years of inactivity, of smoking, drinking, and overeating, who concern me.

Pulse taking involves two stages. To start, everyone sits in a circle and quietly focuses on how to find a normal, nonexercise pulse. It is important to take enough time for this to make sure that everyone has understood the finger placement and has actually found a pulse. The three pulse-taking methods are as follows:

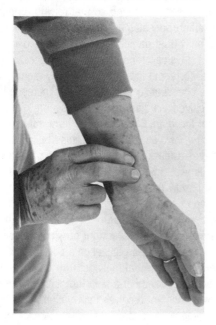

Taking the radial pulse: Figure 3.1 shows the location of the radial artery at the wrist. Place the first three fingers gently between the rather pronounced tendon and the outside edge of the wrist—that's where the

artery is and where you can find the sometimes elusive pulse. Use the pads of your fingers instead of your fingertips, keep the hand and wrist relaxed, and do not apply pressure. Applying pressure can reduce blood flow and make it difficult to feel the pulsation.

Taking the carotid pulse: Look at Figure 3.2 to find the location of the carotid artery at the neck. This

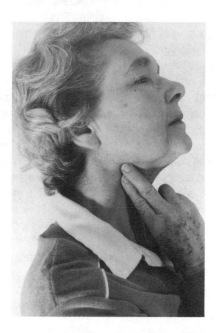

is a larger artery, and although it is easier to pick up the pulsation there, it takes practice to locate. Ask the group not to talk for a few minutes but to concentrate on this task. Have them place the pads of their three first fingers gently over the soft tissues of the neck just below where the jawbone ends. To prevent distorted pulsation, make sure they do not apply pressure. During or after exercise, most people find it easiest to take the pulse at this artery.

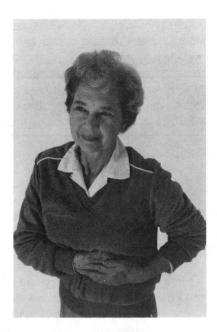

Finding heart rate at the heart: It's hard not to react with panic when you see someone in your class clutching his or her chest near the heart! But for a few, this is the easist method because the heart beat is stronger and clearer than either at the radial or carotid artery. Figure 3.3 shows hand placement: right palm and fingers hug the rib cage where the heart is located; left hand is placed over the right.

All this sounds simple enough, and it is very surprising to discover the variety of problems this seemingly simple task presents. Watching everyone totally engrossed in "listening in on themselves" is fascinating. There is head-shaking ("it just isn't there!"), going from one spot to the next, frowning and worried-looking ("What if I don't have a pulse?") expressions. Finally, a face will light up with recognition: "I found it!!!" Some simply will not be able to find the pulse at rest. The next step then is to have everyone get up and start some vigorous arm swinging and light jogging in place for a few minutes. Then everyone searches again, finding their pulse more quickly and easily because of the short burst of exercise. If someone is still confused, spend some time alone with that person at the end of the class.

The second stage is instructing everyone to count his or her pulse for whatever length of time you determine. In this practice session, I suggest 30 seconds the first time around. I give people the signal to start counting as I look at my watch. When I say "Stop," everything falls apart. Only a few will have an accurate count, which becomes evident from answers to my question, "What number did you come up with?" The range is incredible. Some admit that they lost their concentration, lost count, skipped a few beats here and there, had their pulse suddenly disappear, got too confused, and so on. So we try again, this time for only 15 seconds. The picture looks a little better, but there still is general confusion. I suggest that everyone practice this to perfection at home, both at rest and after climbing a flight of stairs, and come up with a fairly consistent figure for the 15-second count.

Pulse taking is a skill that requires practice, but with patience everyone can learn to become accurate. Over the years only one person in my seniors classes wanted absolutely nothing to do with this pulse taking. She felt very uncomfortable with what she perceived to be "body invasion," listening in on what she thought she had no business listening to, and I could not help her get over this feeling.

During the next class we practice pulse taking while involved in endurance activities. Those who did their homework will come up with their exercise heart rate quickly and accurately. Checking pulse rate *during* exercise is important for knowing what is happening at that specific time, not after sitting down to relax. Heart rate drops very quickly as soon as activity is slowed. Of course, one has to briefly stop and stand still to concentrate on this task. The suggestion is to count for only 10 or 15 seconds because there is an already significant drop after that time. This figure is then multiplied by 6 or 4 to come up with the full minute heart rate. For my seniors, I suggest keeping count for 15 seconds so they do not feel so rushed, then multiplying by 4. A count of between 105 and 130 beats for the minute is a good range for this age group, and anything above 130 means that they are exercising too strenuously and need to slow down. This can be achieved by keeping arm movements a little less enthusiastic, not lifting the knees quite as high when skipping, or slowing down the general pace a bit. *Note:* It is important to know that some heart medications containing Beta blockers cause a generally slowed heart rate. Persons taking such medication should not attempt to bring their exercise heart rate up to the recommended level.

Once everyone has learned the techniques, has practiced both at home and in the classroom, and is confident in doing it right, I do not repeat group pulse taking sessions; however, I encourage individual monitoring if and when each person feels it to be important. I have learned that because pulse taking requires full concentration and is such a different experience for most of the seniors, they do much better on their own.

muscular fitness

Muscular fitness (strength, endurance, and flexibility) can only be brought about and maintained if muscles are put to use. Sitting in rocking chairs requires little effort, and too little effort causes much of the decline in physical ability as we age. We fear this decline when we think of growing older—becoming helpless, dependent and weak, giving up more and more of what we used to be able to do, and needing others to do it for us.

Our society does not encourage older people to continue using their physical abilities. Our vocabulary expressing the common attitudes is not exactly confidence inspiring. We talk about older people who "go down the drain," are "over the hill," "on their last leg," and "past their prime." We expect older folks to "act their age" and "take it easy." Even very real complaints may be shrugged off with comments such as, "Well, you are not as young as you used to be," or, "At your age, what do you expect?" Older people, like everyone else, have the right to feel well and to be strongly supported and encouraged into a lifestyle that enhances this expectation. Instead, we manage to convey in many ways that they should expect to feel worse, to get weak, to become dependent, and to be relegated to observing life rather than participating in it. In our programs, however, we can encourage seniors to develop better cardiovascular endurance and overall muscle strength and flexibility rather than giving up and rusting out. "Use it or lose it" applies to everyone and becomes a crucial concept in the older years.

The term *hypokinetic disease* is used to describe muscular deterioration resulting from disuse. This deterioration can be reversed at any age with well-directed exercise. Being out of shape has nothing to do with getting older but is the result of not exercising. As soon as we commit ourselves to regular activity, we "shape up." Weight lifting is popular not because it makes people younger, but because it makes them stronger. We know

that the muscles underneath abdominal flab can become strong with faithful sessions of daily sit-ups. For muscular weakness to turn into strength, we have to impose demands on muscle groups. The amount of time and energy we spend with strengthening exercises determines the rate of improvement we experience.

These basic principles are true for everyone, including older folks. It is logical that the physical decline so common in aging is greatly influenced by an inactive lifestyle, by moving less and sitting more, by replacing physical work and activity with television watching. It is then also logical to consider the option of reversing at least part of this decline by getting out of the rocking chair and back into a more active way of living.

Muscle strength is gained by "overloading" muscles, and weight lifting will increase strength fastest. But just as it is not reasonable to look at jogging as an appropriate endurance activity for most seniors, lifting weights is not a logical program for muscle strengthening at that age. Basic calisthenic exercises suggested in this guide will result in improved muscle strength for meeting the demands of daily living. Arms and legs strengthen, posture improves, low-back problems diminish, and there is greater protection from muscle and joint injury.

muscular endurance

Muscular endurance is related to strength. It is the muscle group's ability to keep going with a given activity or task over a longer period of time without fatiguing. A hiker's leg muscles need to be strong, but they also need good endurance to keep up this activity for the number of hours it will take to conquer the mountain. Good muscle endurance means that we can do whatever we need or have to do without having to stop because of muscle fatigue. Muscle power is not needed in an older person's life, but adequate muscular strength and good muscle endurance are important for coping with normal work and activities and for getting through the day without exhaustion.

flexibility

Flexiblity is the range of motion possible at a joint and is affected by three factors: the way bones "fit" at a joint, the tightness of the ligaments of the joint, and the elasticity of the muscles associated with the joint. It is the elasticity and length of these tissues surrounding a joint that give us either good range of motion or create the stiffness and lack of flexibility that many people experience. Flexibility is necessary for normal, safe range of motion: for stretching, bending, twisting, turning, lifting, and throwing.

Flexibility helps prevent injuries in different ways. Flexible muscles are less susceptible to tears caused by a sudden stretch. This stretch may simply be bending forward to pick up something from the floor or awkward positioning when making the bed. There is less chance of ligament sprain or joint injury if the joint is flexible enough and has good range of motion. Supple muscles also put less strain on the adjacent joints during physical work and activity. Tight hamstring muscles in the back of the thigh, for example, make persons more prone to injury of these muscles themselves but also put increased stress on the lower back and hips because these muscles are connected.

Sedentary living affects flexibility greatly, as does stress to which muscles in the back of the body respond by tightening and shortening. Too much sitting in poor posture can cause stiffness and pain in neck, shoulders, and upper back. A low level of activity means that joints and muscles are no longer moved through the complete range of motion for which they are constructed, restricting movement patterns. Changes naturally occur in joints, tendons, ligaments, muscles, and connective tissues as we grow older, but these changes are speeded up by doing less and less as the years go by. Stretching and flexibility exercises make a significant contribution to minimizing these changes by keeping muscles and tissues around joints elastic for more youthful movement.

Lack of flexibility affects posture and gait which, even from a distance, can signal that an older person is approaching. Poor posture and shuffling, however, do not have to accompany the aging process. Those who remain strong and flexible will continue to walk and stand erect and keep a youthful bounce in their stride.

body composition

Body composition, the ratio of lean and fat tissue we carry, is one more indicator of fitness and health. Scales, unfortunately, have limited value when it comes to separating lean body mass from fat weight. The term *overweight* is slowly becoming obsolete medically and is being replaced by the more accurate term *overfat*.

It is possible to fit right into the "ideal weight" charts published by life insurance companies and feel smug about not being overweight; however, you may be "overfat," carrying around a much higher percentage of body fat than is healthy. People who do not exercise tend to fall into this category. In contrast, the well-exercised person might exceed the weights suggested on charts and seem overweight but have a low body fat

percentage. Strong, well-exercised muscles weigh more than fat, and it is possible to gain a few pounds as a result of starting a regular exercise program. This weight gain would represent an increase in healthy, metabolically active, lean muscle tissue—the good kind of weight to carry around.

Unfortunately, most adults, weighing the same at age 40 as they did at 20, have gained fat over the years unless they stayed physically active. The average sedentary adult has lost muscle weight and replaced it by fat gained, and bathroom scales cannot tell that story. Researchers use a different type of scale to determine body composition: a large water tank in which the person is submerged while sitting on a special canvas sling chair hanging from what looks like the old-fashioned grocer's scale.

The more fat you have, the more you float, and the less you weigh underwater. In this situation it is not the very fat person who will break the scales: Underwater he will be very light instead. The lean, muscular people weigh more, and they are the healthier ones. The underwater weight is compared to the weight on land, and complex formulas are used to come up with a fairly accurate determination of how much of the total body weight is lean, how much is fat.

If heart, lung, and muscle power decline as we age, it is mostly the result of a much more sedentary lifestyle. The increase in body fat shows a typical imbalance: Calorie intake has not been adjusted to this decrease in activity. The amount of food consumed stays the same, but far fewer calories are burned in physical activity. Thus, the pounds slowly accumulate and muscle weight is replaced by fat weight. Much as we would like to blame spare tires and pot bellies on sluggish metabolism, heredity, glands, or getting older, the simple fact is that we eat too much and move too little as we grow older.

Older people are just as concerned about how they look and feel as younger people. No one enjoys gaining weight and squeezing into tight clothing. Even though perfect measurements are not a reasonable goal in the senior years, lowering body fat and increasing lean muscle, tightening up and trimming down, is possible and realistic. If we help our older students to appreciate the health benefits of such changes, they will be encouraged into better eating and exercise habits.

exercises to avoid

A number of common exercises and activities should be eliminated because they can cause strain and injury. These exercises serve no good purpose in terms of exercise benefits and can be replaced with safer, more effective movements. Let's not get people out of rocking chairs to end up on crutches or in bed!

The toe touch from a standing position is popularly believed to remove an unwanted "pot." This is one of many exercise myths to discard. Especially with knees locked, this forward-bending places great pressure on discs in the lower back. You literally hang by your back ligaments, stressing the spine and sciatic nerve. Forward-bending is a normal movement and helps in retaining back flexibility, but knees should always be comfortably bent to be safe.

Many older people get dizzy on forward-bending (standing or chair-sitting), especially if they come up too fast. Keep head up while bending and come up slowly if prone to dizziness.

Deep knee bends are part of military drills but were condemned by the President's Council on Physical Fitness long ago. All deep knee bend variations overstretch the supportive ligaments around the knee and compress cartilage, making knees susceptible to injury, and permanent damage can result. When overstretched, ligaments, unlike muscles, do not return to their normal length. Knee-bending exercises are great for strengthening quadriceps muscles, but only if knees are not bent below a 90° angle (as if sitting on a chair). Try to keep the knees bent over the ankles so they don't protrude, and don't let buttocks go below knee level in this squatting position. These exercises should not cause discomfort and pressure in knee joints. Demonstrate how to perform these types of movements correctly. Most older folks I know have some problems with their knees, and doing these kinds of exercises incorrectly aggravates the problem.

Straight leg sit-ups can contribute to low back pain by straining back muscles and ligaments and elongating nerves. They also make minimal use of abdominal muscles, involving hip flexors instead. Knees should always be bent during sit-ups to keep the back protected. Unless the older person has kept abdominal muscles in good condition, full sit-ups are a real struggle, and not too many of my older students can do these without undue strain. A quarter sit-up is a more effective exercise: Abdominal muscles can't cheat, and the lower back is not stressed. For these, just the head, shoulders, and upper back curl up from the floor while the fingertips reach for the knees.

Straight leg raises, unless you are in top shape, also place tremendous strain on the lower back. Most people are not strong enough to keep the spine pressed tightly to the floor while both straight legs are raised and lowered. The pelvis will rotate forward, causing the lower back to arch and raise away from the floor, creating a very accentuated sway back and often causing instant pain. This exercise is definitely not appropriate for older persons.

Yoga exercises are for those with extreme flexibility, strongly developed balance, and good muscle strength and control. Yoga positions, such as the Plow, place too much strain on the back and neck and should never be attempted in a seniors' program. Neck vertebrae are not strong enough to support the body's weight. The strain of this position also stresses blood vessels in the brain and causes restricted breathing.

Isometric exercises (tensing one set of body muscles against another or against an immovable object, such as weight lifting or strenuous push-ups) are not safe for older persons, especially for those with high blood pressure or heart conditions. Arterial pressure increases during isometric contractions, and breathing is restricted. Exercises that are rhythmical (those in which muscles alternately contract and relax, or shorten and lengthen) and that allow comfortable, rhythmical breathing are recommended because they increase heart rate and cardiac output, improve cardiovascular and muscular fitness, and maintain flexibility.

Jumping rope requires more endurance and coordination than most seniors are capable of. I use jump ropes in all younger adult classes but hide them from my older students. It's too easy to trip and fall. In addition, repeated jumping is too stressful for aging weight-bearing joints such as ankles, knees, and hips. Comfortable, less forceful endurance activities like brisk walking, light jogging, or skipping are safer and allow everyone to participate safely and without injury.

exercise attire

The changes in exercise clothing over the years have been fun to observe. Initially, women appeared in heels and dresses, skirts and blouses, silk stockings, jewelry, and, of course, girdles. Men came in suit slacks and dress shirts. Somehow it seemed that everyone dressed up for the occasion instead of "dressing down." Convincing the women, most of whom had never owned slacks, to buy an inexpensive but comfortable pair took some time. One older friend's husband steadfastly undermined her attempts to purchase slacks for cold winter days. "It looks too mannish," he would say. "I like my woman in skirts and dresses." Those who finally bought slacks would bring them to class and change there because they didn't feel comfortable being seen in public this way. But those first courageous souls affected the others, and soon everyone wore slacks.

Over the years, class members became more daring, and some bought sweatpants, inspiring others to do the same. When running shoes became popular, I encouraged those who could afford them to buy a reasonably priced pair because good shoes might also encourage regular walking. More recently, everyone appears in comfortable exercise clothing. The group looks sharp in the "Seniors On The Move" T-shirts we had printed.

In warm weather, I suggest wearing shorts and cotton T-shirts. Initially, many were concerned about their "lumpy" legs. But I insist that the focus is on comfort during exercise, not on fashion or on winning a beauty contest. I recommend that everyone wear affordable light-weight sneakers or running shoes. Running shoes need to be safe for indoor use, allowing for safe lateral and twisting movements. Soles should be relatively smooth and not wider than the shoe itself, nor too high. With the discount I arranged at a local sporting goods store, this investment has spurred many into walking more on their own, too.

In winter, people dress in layers, wearing sweaters or lightweight sweatshirts over T-shirts so that they can peel when body temperature rises. Sweatpants have become a favorite piece of clothing, not only in the classroom but also at home. Girdles disappeared long ago and so did jewelry and make-up. Everyone comes prepared for some sweating and a good workout. Clothing is individual, comfortable, and bright, ranging from shades of pinks and purples to aqua and orange. The casual clothing and cheerful colors are invigorating.

Feeling more comfortable in "practical" clothing like shorts or sweatpants with T-shirts, I don't wear leotards for teaching my seniors classes. The general exercise movement's strong focus on "perfect bodies" and the fashion industry's push for sexy leotards and clinging body suits disturbs me. I believe that such attire worn by instructors makes older students too self-conscious by forcing comparison and sets the instructor apart from the group. I also notice that what I wear sets a trend, so I keep my attire unobtrusive, inexpensive, and comfortable. By dressing alike, we are not set apart and can be truly comfortable with ourselves and each other.

exercise equipment to find, make, or buy

A variety of simple, inexpensive hand apparatus is available to enhance any fitness program and make classes more interesting and challenging: Exercises are performed more completely, stretching is more effective, and sociability and interaction through partner and group activities are fostered through this equipment. "Staple exercises" become more creative, and new ideas are easily generated. However, because many seniors programs are limited by tight budgets, equipment usually costs little or nothing, is donated, or is handmade. You may want to speak to some of your local service organizations if you need financial help in setting up a new program or to buy new equipment for an existing one. (We purchased our first record player with money contributed by the Rotary Club.)

wooden dowels

Wooden dowels, or broomsticks, can come from different sources. I make a yearly trip to a broom factory to buy inexpensive broomstick seconds. (They usually have splintered ends that must be sawed off and sanded.) Wooden dowels, 3/4" or 5/8" thick, can be purchased at lumberyards or hardware stores. These dowels tend to be only 36 in. long, which is a little short for anyone with shoulder problems. A 42-inch broomstick allows more comfortable range of motion. A much longer stick can become a dangerous weapon in the classroom. Purchased wooden dowels are quite expensive, but participants will be happy to make a small contribution by buying their own or bringing a broomstick from home. These wooden wands can be easily stored in a garbage can, which can be pulled out of a storage closet.

beanbags

Beanbags are easy to make and store. The sewing circle at our senior center made ours with fabric remnants donated by a local fabric shop. If there is no sewing circle ready to take up the project, you may find volunteer seamstresses in your class. We bought the least expensive bulk beans, converting them into bargain exercise equipment for tossing, catching, improving coordination, and having a lot of fun.

A 5" × 7" beanbag is a good size and should be filled loosely with one-half pound of dry beans. If the bag is filled to the brim, it is hard to hold and becomes a rock-hard weapon when tossed. One beanbag per person is enough. All beanbags can be easily stored in a plastic washbasket.

bicycle inner tubes

Bicycle inner tubes are free for the taking. Go to your local bike shop where they are discarded by the dozens during biking season. Bike inner tubes can be used for a variety of endurance activities, for partner exercising, and for stretching.

First, valves have to be removed. The best tool to use is an Exacto knife. Cut very closely around the valve to keep the hole as small as possible; otherwise, the tube will quickly tear when used. Do not avoid this project; it is easy to get hurt on these metal valves.

upholstery webbing bands

Upholstery webbing bands are my invention, the result of one productive sleepless night. Upholstery webbing is a sturdily woven 2-inch wide cotton band, available at fabric mills or upholstery supply shops. It can be purchased by the yard and is another exercise equipment bargain. Each person requires 7-1/2 yards of this webbing. To make these bands, fold over 8 inches or so at each end of the band for a loop. (Make the loops large enough to fit shoed feet.) Then machine-stitch loops with strong thread, stitching back and forth a number of times so that seams will not open under stress.

This white webbing is quickly restored by washer and dryer when dirty or can be dyed in cheerful colors to add life to the classroom. After use, everyone returns their bands in a tidy roll to my "grab bag" so that I don't have a tangled mess. To your bag of bands, add a number of sturdy 3" metal rings, which you can purchase at hardware stores. These you will need for group work using the bands, one ring for each group of five participants.

These bands are especially helpful to those with poor back and hamstring flexibility. They help with anchoring for stretching, resulting in better body positioning and stability.

scarves

Scarves, too, add life, color, and variety to an occasional class. The women, especially, enjoy creating fluttering patterns; the men are less enthusiastic, even though I remind them that Zorba the Greek danced with a kerchief. (Sturdy, more masculine-looking cotton bandannas appeal more to the men.) Scarves (two per person) are either contributed by class members or made from fabric donated by a willing merchant.

Choose colorful, light, and silky fabrics rather than limp cotton. Light nylons in bright prints look cheerful on a dreary day, and nylon doesn't wrinkle in your storage bag. Cut fabric into napkin-size squares, and if you can find materials that do not ravel, there is no need for seaming the edges.

dumbbells

Small dumbbells (or smartbells, as my students prefer to call them) have to be purchased and, depending on your budget, may have to be low on your list of priorities. Sand weights can be used in their place for upper body strengthening exercises. Ours are 2-lb cast-iron weights, a pair for each participant, and they can be ordered from the factory through your local sporting goods store. (Never hesitate to ask merchants to make prices as low as possible.) These compact little weights are very useful for upper body strengthening and range-of-motion exercises, and we use them often. Our black cast-iron dumbbells look very utilitarian compared to the presently fashionable "Heavyhands" made of shiny chrome with handles, but there is a world of difference in cost, and exercise benefits are the same. Two-pound weights seem to be the most useful for older students. I also have a few sets of one-pounders for those with shoulder problems.

sand weights

Sand weights can be a replacement for these dumbbells if there is no money, and you may have to call on the sewing circle once again. Use sturdy cotton fabrics for the outer pocket, cutting two 8" squares for each weight. Machine-sew three seams of this pocket, leaving one end open to insert a plastic baggy filled with 2 lb of sand. Use fine sand without stones—the kind you find in sand boxes or golf course traps—that can be purchased from construction suppliers or lumberyards. It comes in 50-lb bags and is quite inexpensive, but be sure to let someone with a strong back carry it for you.

You need one pair of sand weights for each person in your class. Storing these is more of a problem than storing beanbags. Thirty sets of weights translate into 120 lb, and you can't pull these out of a storage closet without straining your back. A sturdy dolly arrangement will allow you to wheel a heavy plastic washbasket full of weights around easily.

Make sure that sand is not filled into fabric shells without baggies that are closed with "twistums"; otherwise, the fine sand will sift through and get into everyone's eyes. Ask your seamstresses to sew each seam several times, or they will open easily because of the heavy sand. Hand-stitch the remaining open seam securely.

carpet samples

Carpet samples are adequate exercise mats and easy to stack and store if storage space is limited. I prefer samples with rubber backing because they provide extra cushioning and do not slip around. Carpet samples usually sell for around $2.00, but I have found the local stores willing to make a donation. These contributions create good will and ultimately result in new customers, and as I approach merchants, I make this the selling point.

Even though carpet samples are small, they are long enough to provide padding for all the bony body parts that would suffer most on a hard floor: spine and head, pelvic bones, knees, and elbows. In the back-lying position, it's enough to have the spine and head cushioned, and as you roll over, only the trunk and pelvic area need padding. Those with knee problems need two or even three carpet samples for kneeling exercises to be comfortable.

4
general warm-up and wake-up exercises

I like to begin each class with three sets of warm-up and limbering exercises. Some participants are late risers, still in low gear when they arrive, and need a "body wake-up." Warm-up exercises, however, are important for everyone. They prepare the body for more demanding activities, and we spend as much time as seems necessary before going on to other work. I like to see some perspiration on people's faces. Sweaters and sweatshirts coming off are indicators that warm-ups have been effective. Lively music and vigorous upper body movements help everyone wake up and feel ready for the hour. But there are also days when the overall mood seems more conducive to starting with slow stretching to get overnight kinks out before speeding up a bit.

All major muscle groups and joints should become involved during these first 10 minutes. To minimize fatigue, don't spend more than 15 to 20 seconds with a particular movement before switching to another. Combine several logically progressing warm-up sets, choosing from the variety suggested in this chapter.

Not all exercises described in the following chapters are illustrated. Many of the movements are very basic and easily understood as you read the text. Others are variations of illustrated exercises, and I have made every effort to be clear in my descriptions. Should confusion arise in some instances, your imagination will fill in.

warm-up exercises for the upper body

Set #1: Swimmer's Warm-Up (Stand with feet hip-width apart.)

1 *Crawl Stroke:* Bend forward at waist and swim a vigorous crawl, hips and knees loose. Reach far forward, stretching and limbering up shoulders. Turn to the left and continue, then to the right, and forward again.

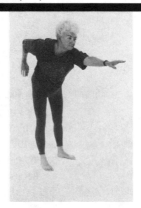 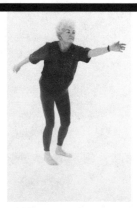

2 *Scissor Arm Swing:* Next is energetic scissor arm swinging, facing forward. Continue while turning upper body to the right, then to the left, and finish facing forward again.

Set #2: Reach and Stretch (Stand with feet hip-width apart.)

1 *Tall Stretch:* Start with hands at shoulders, palms up. Push right arm, then left, toward ceiling. Look up, stretching waistline and lifting rib cage. Push off with light knee bending on each stretch.

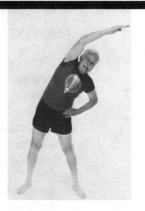 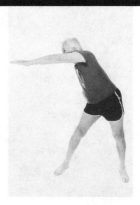

2 *Angle Stretch:* Now reach across face at an angle toward ceiling, arm stretching long each time. Shift weight rhythmically from one foot to the other.

3 *Crossover Stretch:* Reach across at chest level now, arm parallel to floor, to limber waist and lower back.

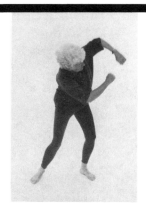

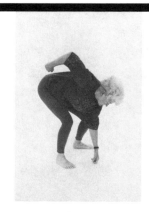

5 Finish with forward crawl stroke; then relax arms and upper body toward floor. Keep knees slightly bent, and let arms swing from side to side, fingertips sliding along floor.

3 *Bent Elbow Arm Swing:* With elbows bent, swing arms briskly from side to side across chest, keeping knees loose.

4 *Floor Punching:* Bend forward, knees bent, and lightly punch fist to floor while other elbow pulls up. While punching, move hips from side to side.

4 *Double Arm Crossover Stretch:* Both arms reach across chest at shoulder level to the right, then to the left. Look at hands as arms stretch long. Continue rocking.

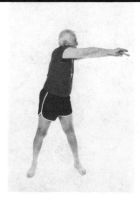

6 Reverse this sequence of movements, ending with tall stretching.

5 *Trunk Twist:* Clasp hands, and extend arms at shoulder level. Smoothly pull arms from side to side and follow this twist with upper body.

Set #3: Twist and Limber (Stand with feet hip-width apart.)

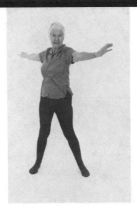

1 *Small Waist Twist:* Bend elbows at shoulder level. Twist upper body right and left, pushing elbow back on each twist, and push off with opposite foot.

3 *Single Arm Fling:* Put left hand on hip. Right arm swings relaxed: across chest over left shoulder, then out wide at right. Repeat several times, looking at hand; then change arms.

2 *Open Arm Waist Twist:* Open arms wide at shoulder level, and continue twisting.

warm-up exercises
for the arms and shoulders

Set #4: Arm Crossing (Stand with feet together.)

1 *Arms Open/Cross:* Bend forward slightly with arms low. Arms open wide, then cross, while knees bend and straighten rhythmically. (Bend when crossing arms; straighten when opening them.)

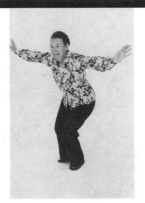 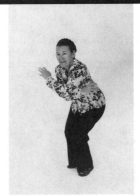

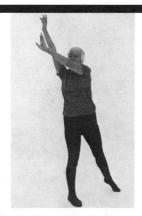

5 *Progression:* Clasp hands and continue double arm fling for stronger waist twist.

4 *Double Arm Fling:* Swing both arms over right, then left shoulder, while shifting weight from one foot to the other.

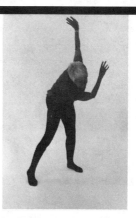

6 *Low Arm Swing:* Bend forward at waist with upper body and arms low. Keep knees loose while arms swing low and relaxed.

2 *Progression:* Continue arm movements, changing from knee-bending to very light, relaxed jumps with feet together.

3 *Progression:* Stay in squat position while arms cross and open. Fingertips drag along floor as arms cross.

4 *Cross and Reach:* As knees bend, arms cross low. As legs straighten, arms open wide and lift overhead. Rise onto toes.

5 *Large Crossing Circles:* Arms cross and circle around in front of chest. Describe large circles, rising onto toes each time wrists cross overhead.

6 *Progression Pattern:* Practice for coordination and fun: Arms cross, open, circle inward and around. Then arms open, cross, circle outward and around. There will be general confusion, but practicing is always fun and good exercise.

7 Shake legs and arms to relax. Using large muscle groups raises the internal thermostat quickly.

Set #5: Shoulder Rolling (Stand with feet together.)

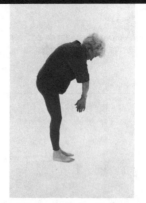
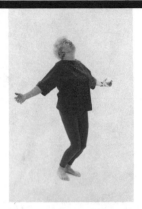

1 *Easy Shoulder Rolling:* Arms down and relaxed. Shoulders push forward, then pull back, hands drawing a figure 8 next to hips. This exercise limbers up shoulders, chest, and shoulder girdle.

2 *Shoulder Rotation:* Extend arms out at shoulder level. Draw a large figure 8, rotating arms for limbering shoulders and toning upper arms.

3 *Energetic Shoulder Rolling:* Continue this movement with more energy and stronger knee movements. Try to involve the whole body. Knees stay loose, and there is move- ment in the pelvis. As arms pull back, knees push forward and pelvis tucks under. This movement feels like a strong wave moving through the body.

Set #6: Arm, Shoulder, and Leg Wake-Up (Stand with feet together.)

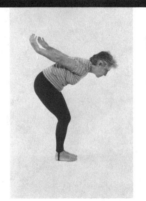

1 *Relaxed Double Arm Swing:* Both arms swing forward and back at sides, loosely and comfortably. Knees are involved, bending and straightening rhythmically.

2 *Low Double Arm Swing:* Continue swinging arms, but bend knees enough to drag fingertips along floor on each downswing to involve thigh muscles.

Set #7: Coordinated Arm Swinging (Stand with feet hip-width apart.)

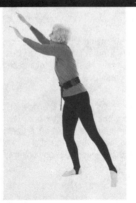
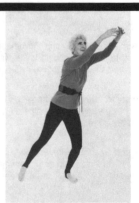

1 *Double Arm Swing and Reach:* Shifting weight from one foot to the other in a rocking motion, swing both arms high at right, reaching toward ceiling, then down and across body high to the left. Bend knees and push off for each swing. Look at hands.

4 *Shoulder Circling:* Keep arms down and relaxed. Pull shoulders up, push them back to bring shoulder blades close, lower them to relax.

5 Finish this set with relaxed shoulder shrugging.

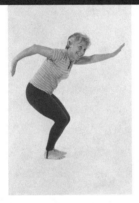

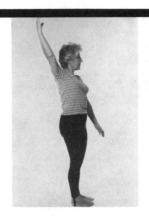

head as it moves up and around. Add light knee bending.

5 *Single Arm Swing and Circle:* Right hand on hip. Left arm swings forward, back, and then circles from front to back twice. The pattern is swing, swing, circle, circle. Repeat with right arm.

6 Finish this set with relaxed double arm swinging. Keep legs involved throughout these movements to warm leg muscles and lubricate knee joints.

3 *Single Arm Reach:* As one long arm reaches forward, other elbow pulls far back, simulating cross-country ski poling. Keep movements soft and rhythmical, upper body forward slightly, and knees loose.

4 *Single Arm Circling:* Stand tall and circle right arm, then left from front to back. Keep circles large for complete range of motion in shoulder joints: arm is straight and close to

2 *Swing and Circle Arms in Place:* Continue swinging arms right, left, and then around in a large circle to the right, up, and around. Finish with arms swinging to the right. Then reverse direction: Swing left, right, and circle to the left and around. Keep rhythm with easy knee bending.

3 *Swing and Circle Moving:* For coordination practice, add a simple side step to this arm movement: Swing arms right, weight onto right foot. Swing left, weight onto left foot. As arms circle to the right, step right with right foot, bring feet together, and again step right (legs are apart again now). Arm pattern is swing, swing, circle; foot pattern is step, together, step. Repeat, stepping to the left. This pattern always causes confusion and needs practicing again each time. It's one of the rare occasions when you might want to turn your back to the class to demonstrate.

4 *Swing and Circle With Light Jumps:* To make this movement a little more vigorous, turn the side steps into light jumps now. Arm movements continue, and the step-together-step movement becomes a light jump-together-jump.

5 Stretch tall and take a deep breath, lower arms and breathe out. Repeat several times while walking around for a minute.

Set #8: Chest Stretching (Stand with feet together.)

1 *Single Arm Lift and Bend:* Start with arms down, hands on thighs. Lift right arm forward and up, close to ear. Push arm back strongly; then bend elbow and touch palm to upper back. Stand erect! Stretch arm up again, then lower it to starting position, and repeat with other arm.

2 *Double Arm Lift:* Raise both arms, straight and high, fingers pointing at ceiling. Push back several times, close to face. Lower arms to relax.

3 *Double Arm Lift and Bend:* Raise arms and push back. Bend elbows and touch palms to upper back, keeping spine erect. Straighten arms up again; then lower them to starting position.

4 *Lateral Single Arm Stretch:* With legs apart and elbows bent at shoulder level, open right arm wide to stretch inner arm and chest muscles, left fingertips at chest. Look at right hand. Bend elbow and repeat with left arm.

5 *Arms Cross and Open:* Cross long, straight arms in front at shoulder level, stretching upper back. Then open wide to stretch chest.

warm-up exercises for the hips and torso

Set #9: Hip Limbering (Stand with feet hip-width apart.)

1 *Hip Swing:* Start with arms down and relaxed. Swing hips briskly from side to side, knees loose, and arms swinging along. Movement comes from hip joints, helping with limbering and lubricating.

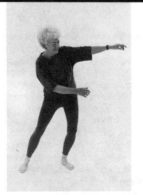

2 *Hip Swing Pattern:* Alternate four fast hip swings with two slow ones, adding a little extra push to these two. Pattern is swing hips right, left, right, left, and then push twice to the right, twice to the left. Knees stay relaxed.

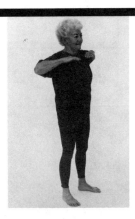 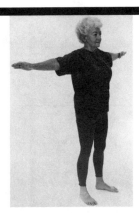

7 Shake arms out; shrug shoulders comfortably.

6 ***Snap and Stretch:*** Push elbows back at shoulder level, feeling upper back muscles contract. Relax elbows forward. Then open arms wide to stretch chest.

3 ***Hoola Hip Swing:*** Raise arms overhead. While hips swing from side to side, slowly lower arms and bend forward to bring hands to floor. Continue swinging hips while straightening up again and bringing arms overhead. Knees stay loose throughout.

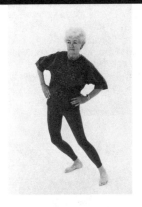 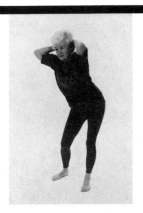

4 ***Hip Circling:*** Hands on hips, rotate hips in large circles to the right several times, then to the left. Keep knees relaxed to allow for greater range of movement. This movement comes from the hip joints, and isolating the hips seems very difficult for many older students. It is helpful to explain and demonstrate first.

5 ***Progression:*** Once mastered, continue this hip circling with hands behind head.

Set #10: More Hip Limbering (Stand with feet together.)

1 *Leg Rotation:* Place ball of left foot on floor, and turn foot inward as far as possible. Then rotate leg from the hip, turning foot and pelvis out. Imagine drilling a hole into the floor. Repeat several times, working at strong movement of hip joint.

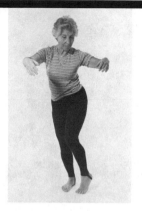
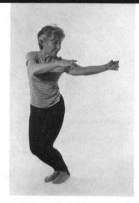

2 *Travel Twist:* Keep feet together, elbows bent at shoulder level. Move sideways, sliding feet along floor: Toes lift and lead to the right; heels lift and follow. A swiveling motion of the hips propels you sideways, and arms move in opposition for balance.

Set #11: Side Bending (Stand with feet more than hip-width apart.)

1 *Easy Side Bending:* Arms are down, hands touching outsides of thighs. Bend directly to side, hand sliding toward knee while other hand slides up along rib cage. Bend right and left slowly, increasing stretch until hand slides to calf level.

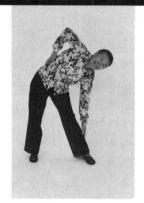
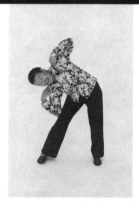

2 *Bending With Shoulder Hold:* Put hands on shoulders. Bend to bring right elbow toward outside of right thigh while left elbow points at ceiling. Look up, and alternate slowly for good stretching.

Set #12: Reach, Twist, and Bend (Stand with feet hip-width apart.)

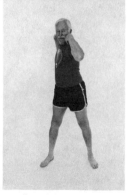

2 *Twist and Bend:* Stay in same starting position. Twist right, bend comfortably toward right leg, and slowly return to upright position. Twist left and bend over left leg. Keep head up.

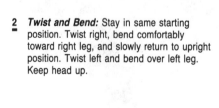
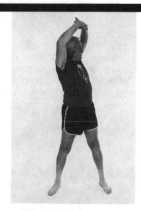

1 *Elbow Leading Twist:* Put hands behind head, spine erect. Twist right and left slowly, pushing elbow back.

3 *Window Twist:* Lift arms overhead, elbows slightly bent, head directly between arms. Twist right and left, looking through arms.

3 *Grapevine Step:* Move sideways with the famous Zorba the Greek grapevine step: Bring left foot across right in front, step right with right foot. Bring left foot across right in back, and again step right with right foot. Continue moving halfway across room before changing direction.

This step, too, takes demonstration, practice, and a little patience. Emphasize moving from the hip, keeping knees relaxed. There is a tendency to keep legs stiff which causes awkward movement. There is so little lateral movement in our daily lives that especially those with poor coordination confront a mental block. You can help those who really find it difficult to catch on by holding their hands and talking them through each step slowly, then using strong hand contact to convey a more relaxed, comfortable way of moving sideways with this step. Everyone learns eventually, and it's worth practicing because this fun step can be included in many of the other activities.

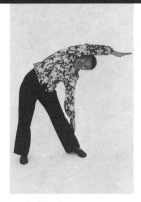 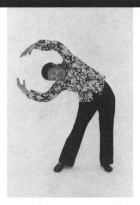

5 *Large Arm Circling:* Clasp hands, and circle upper body to the right. Let fingertips slide along floor and come up from the left. Knees bend on coming down. Circle slowly, three times in each direction.

3 *Bending With Arm Lift:* Continue bending, but slide one hand toward lower leg, other arm raised overhead, close to face.

4 *Double Arm Side Bending:* Lift arms overhead, elbows slightly bent. Bend from side to side, adding a gentle bounce to each stretch.

4 *Window Twist and Bend:* Keep arms overhead and turn upper body to the right. Then bend over right leg to touch hands to foot. Keep knee relaxed to avoid low back strain. Straighten up with arms overhead, twist to the left, and bend to touch left foot.

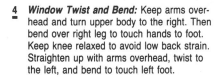 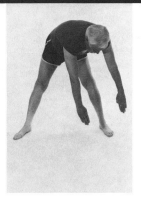 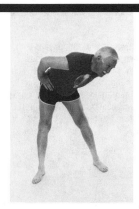

5 *Trunk Circling:* Hands on hips, circle upper body to the right several times, then to the left. Move slowly to avoid dizziness.

Set #13: Forward and Back Bending (Stand with feet hip-width apart.)

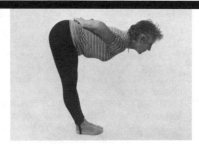

1 *Straight Back Forward Bending:* Put hands behind lower back. Bend forward with chin up, back flat, and legs straight. Bounce gently several times, then straighten up, and bend back a little to look up.

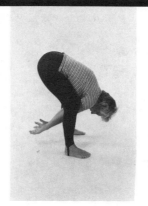 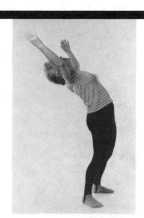

3 *Forward Bending Progression:* Relax upper body forward and reach through relaxed legs for a greater back stretch. Return to upright position and lift arms up into a wide V while bending back slightly to look up.

5 *All-Around Bending:* Bend forward with relaxed knees and reach through legs. Straighten up, arms relaxed at sides, and pause for a moment before bending to the right. Straighten again, place hands on hips, and bend back comfortably. Straighten again; then bend to the left. Circle slowly several times, adding an extra bounce to each movement. Change direction.

6 Finish with upper body and arms hanging forward, knees loose, and body relaxed.

2 *Round Back Forward Bending:* Relax arms, and bend forward. Touch hands to floor, keeping spine round and knees relaxed. Straighten up and bend back slightly; push pelvis forward and place hands on backs of thighs for support. Add a gentle, relaxed bounce to each movement. Alternate slowly to avoid dizziness.

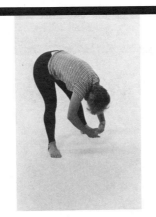 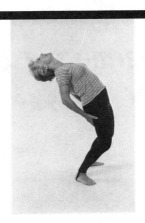

Cont.

4 *Wide Arm Forward Bending:* Hold arms out at shoulder level. Bend forward at waist, chin up, back flat, legs straight, and arms open wide. Gently bounce chest toward floor several times, stretching hamstring muscles.

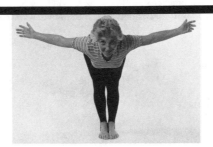

warm-up exercises for the legs and lower back

Set #14: Arm/Leg Coordination (Stand with feet together.)

<u>1</u> **Touch Step:** Lightly touch ball of right foot to floor in front, return foot to center, and touch left foot in front. Arms swing in scissor movement in opposition to foot pattern.

<u>2</u> **Cross Step:** Change pattern. Right foot steps across left foot in front while both arms swing to the right for balance. Then step with left foot across in front of the right, and swing arms to the left.

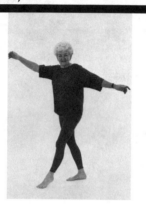

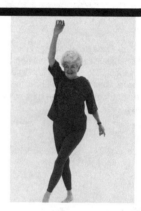

<u>3</u> **Cross Step With Arm Reaching:** As right foot steps across to the left, the left arm stretches at an angle toward the right, and the right arm pulls back, creating a twisting movement at the waist. Look at the hand that reaches forward.

Set #15: Knee and Leg Lifting (Stand with feet together.)

<u>1</u> **Knee to Chest:** Stand erect. Bring one knee up, pulling it close to chest with both hands. Return foot to floor, bring other knee up.

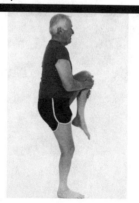

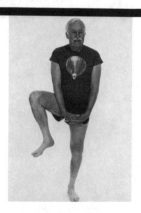

<u>2</u> **Knee to Shoulder:** Keep arms low, and clasp hands. Stand erect, and pull right knee up and out toward right shoulder. Return foot to floor, and pull left knee up toward left shoulder.

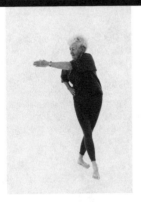

5 Finish the set with easy touch-stepping forward, moving around room now to turn this step in place into a walk. Arms swing relaxed in opposition for balance.

4 *Cross Step With Side Bending:* Continue cross stepping. As right foot steps across, left arm reaches overhead. Bring right arm behind lower back while bending to the right. Change rhythmically, bending right and left.

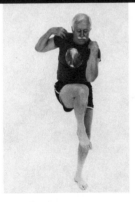

4 *Crossover Leg Kick:* Extend arms out at shoulder level. Kick straight right leg across body, touching foot to left hand. Return foot to floor; then kick across with left leg.

5 *Crossover Windup Kick:* Keep same arm position. Kick right leg across with a low, easy motion. Return foot to floor, and kick same leg high to touch foot to left hand. Change legs.

3 *Knee to Opposite Elbow:* Put hands on shoulders. Bring right knee up and across, turning upper body to the right, and touch left elbow to right knee. Return foot to floor, and touch right elbow to left knee.

Set #16: Forward Kicking (Stand with feet together.)

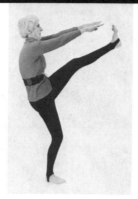
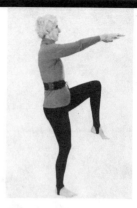

1 *Forward Kick:* Hold arms forward at shoulder level. Kick right leg, then left, up to touch hands. Stand erect.

2 *Knee Lift Forward Kick:* Keep same arm position. Raise right knee toward chest, return foot to floor, and kick leg straight up to bring foot to hands. The knee lift is a little windup for an enthusiastic high kick.

Set #17: Foot and Ankle Warmup (Stand with feet together.)

1 *Jog in Place:* This is a nice rolling movement, and feet keep contact with floor. Roll from heel to ball of foot, shifting weight from one foot to the other. Maintain good posture, keeping arms relaxed.

2 *Toe/Heel Touch:* Hands on hips, bring right leg forward. Keep knee locked while pointing and flexing foot: big toe, then heel touches the floor. Shake legs out; they will be tired.

3 *Foot In and Out:* Hands on hips. Turn right foot in, then out, rotating leg from the hip. Repeat with left foot.

4 *Foot Circling:* Lift right foot away from floor, knee bent. Moving ankle only, rotate foot several times inward, then outward. Change legs; then shake them out to relax.

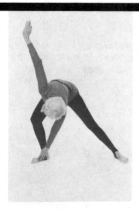
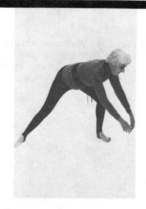
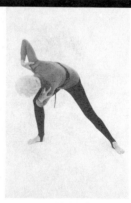

4 *Crossover Toe Touch:* Bend forward, arms out. Shift weight to right leg while touching left hand to right foot. Pull right arm back. Shift weight to left leg, and touch right hand to left foot.

5 *Toe Touch Progression:* Arms and upper body hang forward loosely. Shift weight from one leg to the other, touching weighted foot with both hands each time.

6 *Elbow to Opposite Knee:* Shift weight while trying to touch elbow to opposite knee. This requires a twisting movement at the waist. Those with "spare tires" may not be able to touch but can aim in the general direction.

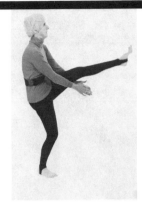

3 *Leg Kick With Hand Clapping:* Extend arms out at shoulder level. Kick right leg forward and clap hands under knee. Return foot to floor while arms open wide again. Alternate legs.

4 *March in Place and Kick:* Hands on hips, raise knees to waist level for three energetic marching steps in place. Every fourth count, kick one leg forward, alternating the kicking leg.

Set #18: Weight Shifting (Stand with feet more than hip-width apart.)

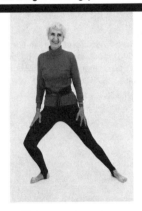

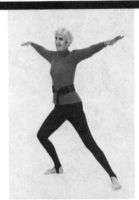

3 *Sustained Weight Shifting:* Shift weight to right thigh, gently bounce four times, shift weight to left thigh, and bounce.

1 *Basic Weight Shifting:* Toes turned out slightly, put hands on thighs, keeping upper body erect. Bend right knee to shift weight onto right leg. Return to starting position, and shift weight to left leg.

2 *Weight Shift Progression:* Arms out, stay in erect posture. While shifting weight, reach far out with extended arm and look at hand.

Cont.

Instructions should be general enough to allow for individual abilities: "Bring elbow *toward* knee" gives the general direction. "Try to touch" gives everyone equal opportunity to try without feeling unsuccessful.

Set #19: Weight Shift With Side Bending (Stand with feet far apart.)

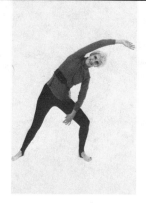
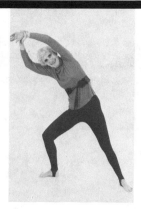

1   *Side Bending:* Bend left knee, placing lower left arm on thigh. Raise right arm and bring it close to ear. Bend to the left for four easy bounces, and look at ceiling for a good stretch. Stand upright and change.

2   *Progression (Side Bending #1):* In stretch position with right knee bent, hold left wrist with right hand and pull against arm to increase stretch. Hold for four easy bounces, and change.

Set #20: Knee Bending (Stand with feet together.)

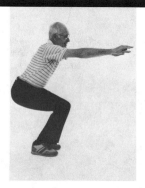
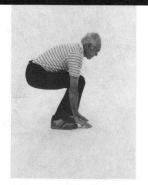

3   *Sustained Knee Bend:* Stay in squat position, hands close to floor, and bounce 10 times to place more sustained demand on thigh muscles. Stretch tall and repeat.

1   *Half Knee Bend:* Hold arms overhead. Bend knees to a 90° angle. Arms stretch forward at shoulder level for balance, and heels stay down. Return to upright position, arms overhead.

2   *Half Knee Bend With Toe Touch:* Arms overhead, stretch tall. Bend knees, this time rounding spine and touching hands to floor. Straighten up and stretch tall again.

Set #21: Leg and Hip Movements With Chair Support

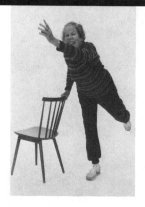

1   *Leg Swing:* Stand sideways behind chair, hand on chair back. Outside leg swings forward and back like a pendulum. Stay in erect posture, keep knee relaxed, and slowly increase height of swing.

2   *Leg and Arm Swing:* This is a coordination teaser, so get into position first: right hand on chair back, left leg forward, left arm back. Swing arm and leg in opposition. As leg swings back, bring upper body forward a little, following outstretched arm.

3   *Knee Up/Leg Swing:* Continue standing sideways. Bring outside knee toward chest, then straighten leg behind you as it swings back. Spine rounds as knee comes toward chest. Look up when leg swings back.

3 *Progression (Side Bending #2):* Arms overhead. Hold hands, palms facing up. Shift weight to the right leg and bend to the right. Bounce four times, keeping head directly between arms, with weight solidly on right foot. Return to starting position and stretch to the left.

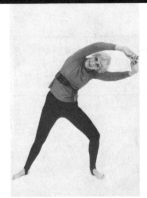

4 Shake legs and arms out to relax.

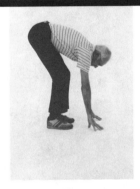

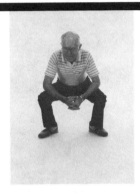

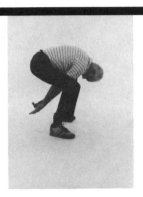

4 *Knees Bend and Straighten:* In half knee bend, fingertips on floor, raise hips and try to straighten legs. Bend and straighten several times while fingertips stay in contact with floor.

5 *Camper's Squat:* Legs apart, turn toes out slightly. Bend knees, and place lower arms on thighs, hands and wrists relaxed. Bounce 10 times in this position, straighten legs to relax, and repeat once more.

6 *Wood Chopper:* Stand with legs apart and hold hands overhead. Swing arms through open legs, bending knees and rounding spine. Return to upright position and repeat several times, swinging arms with enthusiasm. Increase swing, trying to touch hands to buttocks.

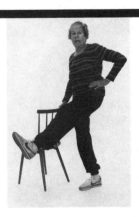

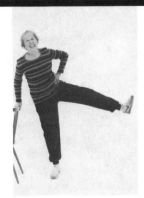

5 *Leg Circling:* Draw a circle with outside leg, increasing circle size to involve hip joint and buttock muscles more.

4 *Leg Swing Forward and Out:* Stand erect. Swing outside leg forward, return to center, then out to waist level, and back to center several times.

Set #22: Spine Limbering With Chair Support

1 *Cat Back:* Face chair seat with hands grasping side edges. Stand 2 ft away from chair. Round the spine, pulling abdominals up and lowering head. Then lift head and straighten spine.

2 *Chair Step-Ups:* Place hands on chair back. Raise right knee, and touch ball of foot lightly to front edge of chair seat. Weight stays on standing foot. (This is not an attempt to climb up onto the chair.) Return foot to floor and step up with left foot.

3 *Hip Wagging:* Stand behind chair, hands on chair back. Step away, stretching arms and spine long. Move hips from side to side, limbering lower back and hip joints, stretching arms, shoulders, and back muscles. Movement comes from hip joints only.

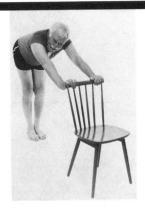

5 *Calf Stretch:* Adjust the long back stretch to include heelcords and calves by pulling toes up and standing on heels. Do not bounce. This is a strong stretch in the lower leg.

4 *Long Back Stretch:* Stay in above position, push hips far back, and keep legs together and straight. Bounce chest toward floor gently several times.

5

exercises using hand equipment

wooden dowels

Set #1: Standing Stretches

1 *Arm Raising:* Stand with legs together, hands shoulder-width apart. Bring dowel overhead, rise onto toes, stretch very tall, and inhale. Lower arms and heels; exhale. Repeat several times.

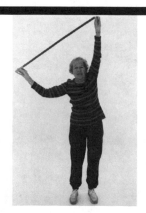

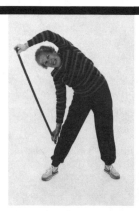

2 *Tall Stretch:* Legs together, hold dowel overhead. Stretching tall, push right end of dowel, then left, toward ceiling.

3 *Tall Side Bending:* Legs well apart, hold dowel overhead. Bend upper body to the right, and try to touch end of dowel to outside of lower leg. Slowly straighten; then bend to the left.

Set #2: Bend and Twist

1 *Bent Elbow Twist:* Stand with legs apart. Bring dowel behind shoulder blades and twist, adding an extra bounce for waistline limbering.

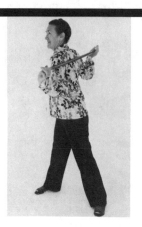

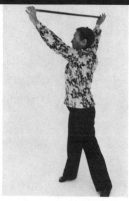

2 *Easy Twist:* Hold arms overhead, head between straight arms. Twist upper body, looking through arms at wall behind you.

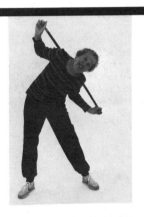

5 ***Trunk Circling:*** With dowel behind shoulder blades, slowly circle upper body to the right several times, then to the left.

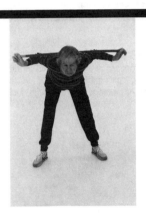

4 ***Side Bending:*** Place dowel behind shoulder blades. With legs well apart, bend slowly from side to side. Push against end of dowel and look at ceiling.

6 ***Flat Back Stretch:*** Stop circling and stay in forward-bent position, legs straight, back flat, and chin up. Gently bounce chest toward floor several times.

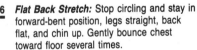

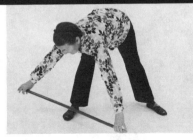

4 ***Waist Twist, Arms Long:*** Bring dowel forward at shoulder level, and hold it with outstretched arms. Continue twisting, keeping arms long, and follow movement with head and upper body.

3 ***Twist and Bend:*** Keep same arm position. Turn upper body to the right, bend over right leg, and touch dowel to foot, bending knee a little. Straighten up, turn to the left, and bend over left leg.

Set #3: Reach, Bend, and Twist

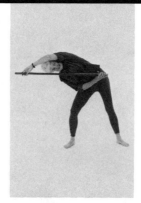

1 *Dowel Push-Away:* Stand with legs apart and dowel held at chest level. Push dowel far over to the left, upper body following arms. Bring elbows in; then push far over to the right.

3 *Shoulder Limbering:* With arms low, lift dowel overhead. Then touch shoulder blades. Straighten arms overhead again and lower them to starting position.

2 *Arm Crossover:* Hold dowel at chest level. Raise left arm out and overhead while right arm pushes across lower body to bring dowel parallel to floor again. Straighten up slowly, and bend to the left.

Set #4: Leg Kicking

1 *Forward Kick:* With legs together, hold dowel forward at shoulder level. In erect posture, kick right leg, then left, up to touch dowel. Alternate with enthusiasm, kicking high.

2 *March in Place and Kick:* Hold dowel in the same position. March in place for three steps, kicking high on fourth.

3 *Coordinated Leg Kick:* Hold dowel forward. Kick right leg up to dowel; then raise arms overhead as foot returns to floor. Lower dowel to chest level as left leg kicks, and raise arms again as leg lowers.

Set #5: Fancy Steps and Kicks

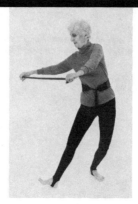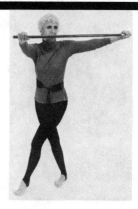

1 *Heel Touch:* Hold dowel forward at shoulder level. Touch right heel to floor, turning foot and pelvis out, and swing dowel to the right. Return foot to center; then touch left heel to floor and swing dowel to the left.

2 *Crossover Step:* Left foot steps across the right in front, ball of foot lightly touching down. Dowel swings to the right, in opposition to foot movement, for balance. Return to center and change.

4 *Round Back Forward Bending:* Keep dowel behind shoulder blades. With legs apart, slump forward, head hanging and back round. Knees stay relaxed.

4 *Knee Up and Kick:* Keep forward arm position, erect posture. Stand with legs together. Bring right knee toward chest, return foot to floor, and kick leg forward to touch dowel. Alternate legs for this windup kick.

3 *Crossover Knee Lift:* Swing dowel to the right while pulling right knee up and across toward left elbow. Return foot to floor and swing dowel to the left, left knee up toward right elbow.

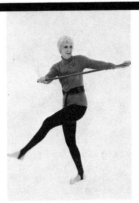

5 *Windup Kick:* Combine the last two movements: Pull knee up and across, put foot down, and kick leg across. Alternate legs, arms moving in opposition.

Combine these five movements into one continuous set to work on coordination.

4 *Crossover Leg Kick:* Continue arm pattern while legs kick across: Left leg kicks to the right as arms swing left.

Set #6: Knee Bending

1   **Bend and Stretch:** Hold arms overhead, legs together. Bend knees to a 90° angle, and touch dowel to floor. Straighten legs and raise dowel overhead.

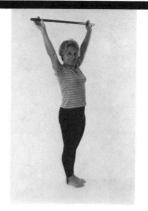

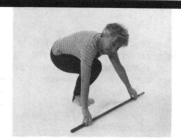

Set #7: More Fancy Steps

1   **Toe Touch Right and Left:** Hold dowel forward at shoulder level. With weight on left foot, touch ball of right foot to floor at right while dowel swings to left. Bring right foot in and step out with left foot, swinging dowel to right.

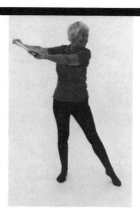

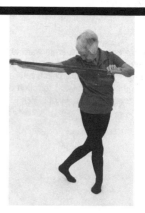

2   **Grapevine Step:** Practice the grapevine step with dowel forward at shoulder level, keeping knees loose and swiveling hips while dowel balances, moving in opposition.

Set #8: Floor-Sitting Abdominal Exercises

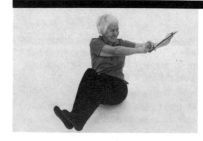

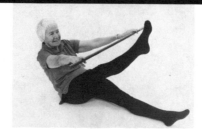

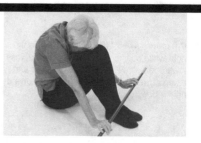

1   **Bent Knee Swing:** Sit with knees bent, feet on floor, arms extended forward. Lift both feet and swing legs to the right; heels touch floor while arms swing to the left. Reverse movement, swinging arms to the right and legs to the left.

2   **Straight Leg Kick:** Keep legs straight and together. Lean back a little, arms stretched forward. Contract abdominals. Kick one leg up and touch foot to dowel. Alternate legs.

3   **Stretch and Curl:** Keep legs together and straight with arms overhead, and stretch tall. Then pull knees close to body, rounding spine, and touch dowel to feet. Extend legs on floor and bring dowel overhead again.

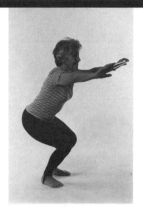

3 *Progression:* Hold arms overhead. Bend knees, and bring dowel down behind back to touch shoulder blades. Stretch tall with arms overhead and legs straight. Again, bend knees and touch dowel to feet; then straighten legs and stretch tall.

2 *Coordinated Knee Bending:* Hold arms overhead. Bend knees, and bring arms forward at shoulder level. Straighten legs and raise arms overhead. Bend knees again, this time touching dowel to floor. Straighten up and bring dowel overhead.

3 *Step-Together-Kick:* Step right with right foot; bring left foot to right. Step right again with right foot, and kick left leg across while dowel swings to the left. The pattern is step, together, step, kick. This takes some practice but is fun to learn. To avoid confusion, turn your back to the class while demonstrating. Alternate stepping to the right, then to the left.

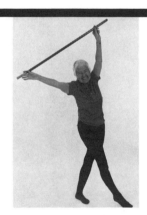

4 *Progression:* Continue this leg work but hold dowel overhead. As leg kicks across, lightly bend upper body in opposition.

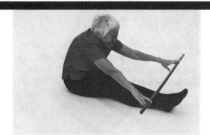

4 *Toe Touch/Lean Back:* With legs straight and together, hold dowel overhead. Bend forward to touch toes. Sit erect again, dowel high. Now lean back, chin close to chest, and touch dowel to thighs. Repeat several times.

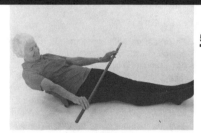

5 *Leg Raise:* Lie on your back with dowel held overhead. Raise right leg and upper body away from floor, trying to touch lower leg or foot to dowel. Return to floor and repeat, raising left leg now. Many participants will find this difficult; encourage them to do what they can.

6 *Dowel Rolling:* Lie on your back with dowel on thighs, fingertips on dowel. While curling up from floor, slowly roll dowel toward knees to sit up. Tuck chin close to chest, and keep spine round as you curl back to floor, rolling dowel toward body.

7 *Buttock Walk:* Sit with dowel held forward. Try to "walk" forward on buttocks, raising one buttock at a time while arms help with balance. Try to "walk" back.

beanbags

Set #1: Shoulder Flexibility

1 *Zipper Opener:* This is something we have practiced often since one class member told us that she always has to wait for the mailman to help her open or close her zipper. Stand with legs together, beanbag in right hand. Bring right hand over right shoulder, left hand behind lower back. Reach up along spine with left hand while right hand pushes down from above. Try to find a corner of the beanbag with the left hand for the change-over and repeat, bringing left hand over left shoulder now. Those with shoulder problems may have to drop the beanbag from upper to lower hand, holding palm open for the catch.

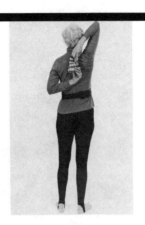

2 *Beanbag Swinging:* With legs together, hold beanbag in right hand. Swing beanbag back, bending knees, then forward and up as legs straighten, and take it overhead with left hand. Left arm now swings back, then forward and up for the change-over.

3 *Single Arm Swing and Circle:* Stand with legs together, put left hand on hip. Hold corner of beanbag in right hand. Swing arm forward, back, and circle around from front to back twice. Repeat several times, keeping rhythm with knee bending. Change arms.

Set #2: Bending and Stretching

1 *Knee Bending:* With legs together and arms overhead, hold beanbag. Bend knees, and place beanbag on floor in front of feet. Stretch tall again without beanbag. Bend once more, pick beanbag up, and lift it high. Repeat several times, concentrating on sequence.

2 *Progression:* With legs together, hold beanbag overhead. Bend knees and place beanbag on floor. While stretching tall again, take a small step to the right with right foot to bring legs apart. With legs apart, bend knees to pick beanbag up. While lifting it overhead, bring right leg back to center so legs are together again for the next kneebend. Repeat, stepping out with left leg.

3 *Beanbag Catch:* Stand with legs together. Toss beanbag up with right hand and catch with left hand, bending knees on the catch. Straighten legs while tossing beanbag up with left hand; bend knees as right hand catches it. Try tossing a little higher each time.

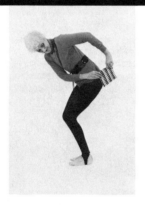

5 *Wood Chopper:* Stand with legs apart. Hold corners of beanbag with both hands. Swing arms through legs, knees relaxed, and touch beanbag to buttocks. Return to upright position, bend elbows, and touch beanbag to upper back. These are vigorous swinging movements.

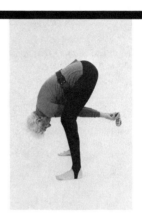

4 *Double Arm Swing:* With legs together, hold beanbag overhead with both hands. Bending knees, swing arms down along outside of right leg, upper body twisting as you look at hands. Swing arms overhead, then down along left leg.

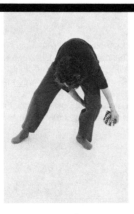

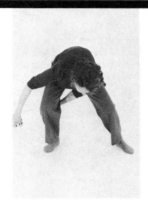

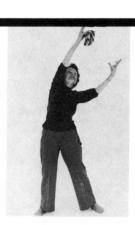

4 *Weight Shifting:* With legs apart and toes turned out slightly, hold beanbag in right hand. Bend forward, and bring beanbag behind left calf, bending left knee. Take beanbag with left hand, and bring it behind right calf, shifting weight to right leg. Continue handing beanbag from one hand to the other in a figure-8 pattern.

5 *Side Bending:* With legs apart, arms out at shoulder level, and palms up, hold beanbag in right hand. Bend to the left, right arm reaching overhead and toward left hand. Place beanbag into open left palm, and bend to the right now.

Set #3: Finger Exercises

1 **Kneading:** Hold beanbag in both hands for vigorous kneading to use all finger joints.

2 **Palm Rubbing:** Place beanbag between open palms. Rub briskly for a good hand massage.

3 **Single Hand Squeeze:** Take beanbag into one hand and squeeze it hard several times. Then change hands.

As suggested earlier, beanbags are easiest to work with if they are not filled too generously. They might burst with these kneading and squeezing actions.

4 **Toss High and Higher:** Toss and catch beanbag with both hands.

5 **Under-the-Knee Toss:** Raise right knee, beanbag in right hand. Toss beanbag from outside under knee and straight up. Catch with both hands. Alternate legs. Start with low tossing, and go a little higher each time. Work on a straight toss to avoid collisions with others.

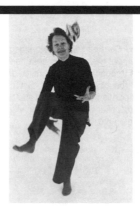

6 **Walk and Toss:** Toss and catch beanbag while walking across room. Then try to toss and catch it while doing polka steps, but be careful not to collide with each other. Place beanbag on head and walk very erect. Walk on toes.

3 **Foot to Foot:** With legs apart, hold beanbag with both hands. Push forward as far as possible. Now slide beanbag along floor to right heel, then to left heel, upper body following arms.

4 **Stretch and Bend:** With legs together, hold beanbag in both hands overhead. Bend forward at a slight angle, touching beanbag to floor next to right foot. Return to tall sitting position, and bend toward left foot.

5 **Impossible Stretch:** With legs together, hold beanbag next to right thigh with right hand. Push beanbag along floor toward feet. Try to slide beanbag around both heels and take it with left hand. Repeat, going from left to right. Most everyone has to cheat by bending knees to get around feet.

Set #4: Tossing

1 **Toss and Catch:** Toss beanbag straight up with both hands. Then catch and "absorb" the beanbag with a light kneebend. Now toss it a little higher, and clap hands once before catching. Toss it higher still, and clap hands twice before catching.

2 **Right and Left Toss:** Toss and catch beanbag with right hand several times, then with left hand. Try for more height.

3 **Toe Touch:** Toss beanbag high, quickly bend knees to touch hands to floor, and straighten up to catch beanbag.

Set #5: Stretching, Floor-Sitting

Cont.

1 **Straddle Stretch:** Sit with legs comfortably apart, both hands on beanbag between legs. Slowly push beanbag forward along floor, chin up. Stretch arms and back long; then return to sitting upright.

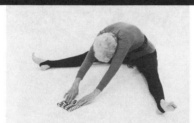 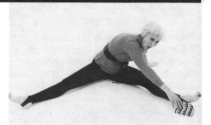

2 **Alternate Leg Stretch:** Sit with legs apart, beanbag on floor, right hand on beanbag. Slide it along inside of left leg, chin up, back long and flat, and aim for ankle. Slide it back and change, left hand pushing along inside of right leg.

Cont.

6 **Beanbag Lift:** Hold beanbag between feet and bend knees. Lean back, hands on floor behind hips. Straighten legs up and bend knees 10 times without dropping beanbag.

dumbbells or sand weights

Set #1: Upper Body Strength

1 *Arm Lifting Series:* Stand erect, legs together, buttocks and abdominals contracted to stabilize lower back. Hold one weight in each hand for eight repetitions of each movement:

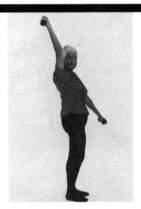 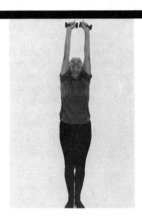

a) Raise straight right arm forward and up; lower slowly. Raise and lower left arm. Stop each lift at ear level.

b) Raise and lower both straight arms. *LIFT*, don't swing.

Set #2: Upper Body Strength

1 *Chest Stretch:* With elbows bent at shoulder level and hands at chest, open arms wide, contracting buttocks to prevent low back arching. Bend elbows and return hands to chest. Focus on deep, rhythmical breathing: Inhale as arms open, and exhale as elbows bend.

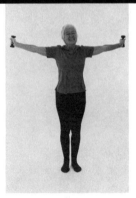

2 *Arms Cross and Open:* Extend straight arms forward at shoulder level. Open arms wide; then cross in front. Focus on contracting buttocks to stabilize lower back.

c) Begin with arms down. Raise both arms out and overhead, stretching tall, and inhale. Lower arms and exhale. To stretch waist and ribcage, improve posture awareness.

d) Combine b) and c). Raise both arms forward and up; lower them. Raise arms out and overhead; lower them.

Working with weights is tiring. Deep breathing is necessary to bring needed oxygen to working muscles. Alternate lifting with relaxed arm swinging to avoid overexertion. Exercises are made easier by sitting on chairs.

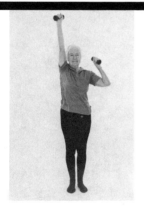

4 *Progression:* Repeat, raising and lowering both arms.

3 *Single Arm Push:* With elbows bent and hands at shoulders, push right arm toward ceiling. Return hand to shoulder as left arm pushes high, and alternate rhythmically. Look up and stretch tall.

Set #3: Arm and Upper Back Strength

<u>**1**</u>   *Touch Front and Back:* Stand with legs together, arms down. Bring weights together in front, then behind back, keeping arms tight and straight.

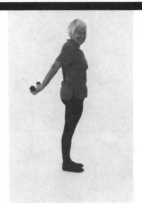 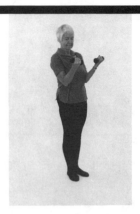

<u>**2**</u>   *Arms Push Away:* Stand erect with arms down, palms facing back. Keep arms straight and close to body, and push them back with small bounces.

<u>**3**</u>   *Bicep Curl:* With arms down and palms facing forward, touch backs of hands to thighs. Keep elbows in contact with waist. Bend elbows and bring weights to shoulders. Slowly lower weights, and repeat 10 times.

Set #4: Arm Swinging to Relax Arms and Loosen Shoulders

<u>**1**</u>   *Scissor Swing:* Stand with legs together. With rhythmical knee bending, swing one arm forward, the other back, in scissor movement.

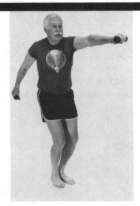

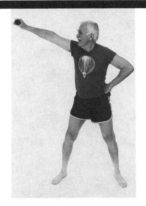

<u>**4**</u>   *Double Arm Side Swing:* Repeat this movement, swinging both arms from side to side. Bend forward a little, knees relaxed; then swing arms lower to stretch back muscles.

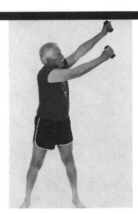

<u>**3**</u>   *Single Arm Side Swing:* With legs apart, put left hand on hip. Extend right arm at shoulder level. While shifting weight from one foot to the other, swing arm down and across to shoulder level at left and back again several times. Repeat with left arm.

4 *Large Arm Circles:* Stand erect, legs together. Alternating arms, slowly circle from front to back, working at large circles for complete range of motion in shoulders. Keep arms close to face.

5 *Arms Pull Away:* Place one weight on floor. Hold other weight behind hips with both hands. Straighten arms and stand very erect, feeling shoulders pull back. Now pull straight arms away from body without bending forward, and inhale. Hold for a few seconds, relax arms, and exhale. Repeat several times.

6 Put weights down and shake arms out; shrug shoulders to relax.

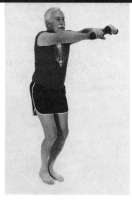

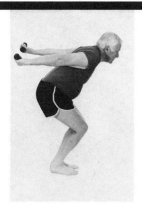

2 *Double Arm Swing:* Swing both arms forward and back very loosely. Continue rhythmical leg movement.

5 *Arms Cross and Open:* With legs apart, cross and open arms wide, being careful not to have weights collide in midair. Add easy knee bending.

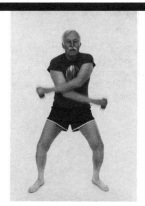

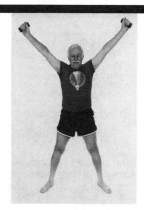

Set #5: Side Bending

1 *Easy Bending:* With legs well apart, relax arms at sides. Bend right and left, allowing weight to pull hand toward floor.

2 *Arm Overhead:* To increase stretch, bend right, right arm hanging loosely. Slowly raise left arm out and overhead, and bring it close to ear. Hold for a few seconds. Repeat, bending to the left.

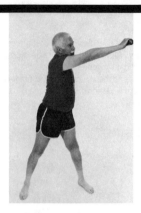

3 *Single Arm Crossover:* With legs apart, push right arm across chest to left, twisting at the waist, and follow with upper body. Now push left arm across to the right. Shift weight from one foot to the other.

Set #6: Knee Bending and Stretching

1 *Double Arm Touchdown:* Bend knees, and touch both weights to floor next to feet. Straighten legs, and raise arms overhead to stretch.

2 *Wide Arm Lift:* Bend knees to touch weights to floor; then straighten legs and raise arms into a wide V.

3 *Half Knee Bend/Arms Cross and Open:* Begin with legs together, arms low. Bend knees, and stay in this squatting position while arms cross, then open wide. Avoid collision of weights.

Set #7: Front-Lying Position

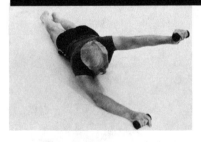

2 *Arc Lifting:* Arms stay forward. Raise right arm, and bring it through the air to rest along lower body. Follow with left arm. Return right arm forward; follow with left arm. Keep chin low.

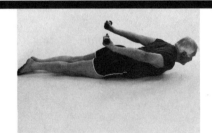

1 *Arm Raise:* Lie face down, arms extended straight ahead. Alternate raising right, then left, arm away from floor, keeping head low to prevent low back arching. Lifting arms just a few inches is enough to help strengthen shoulder girdle and upper back muscles.

3 *Upper Arm Toner:* Lie with arms along body, palms up, chin on floor. Lift both arms, keeping them straight and close to body while pushing toward ceiling.

4 *Large Arm Circles:* With legs together and arms down, cross wrists in front of thighs while bending knees. Bring arms up and around, crossing at chest, and push up onto toes as wrists cross overhead.

4 Put weights down and shake arms, shrug shoulders to relax tired muscles.

4 *Side Arm Raise:* Extend arms out at shoulder level, palms up. Raise arms and chin, and push arms up as if flying with heavy wings.

5 *Chest Stretch:* Put one weight on floor. Hold other weight behind back with both hands. Straighten arms. Raise head and chest while pulling straight arms away from body. Hold for a few seconds; then lower body and arms to relax.

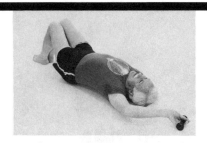 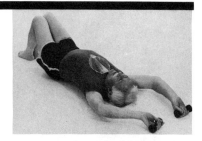

6 *Waist Stretch:* Roll onto back. Bend knees, feet on floor, arms along body with palms down. Bring right arm through the air and overhead to rest on floor close to face. As right arm lowers, left arm is raised overhead. Continue to alternate, reaching high with each arm.

7 *Progression:* Slowly raise both arms overhead, lowering them close to ears. Let weights stretch shoulders, rib cage, and waist. Inhale when raising arms; exhale when lowering.

Set #8: Leg and Abdominal Strength, Floor-Sitting Position

These exercises can be performed only if you have sand weights. Sit and place the 2-lb sand weight over one ankle. Lean back slightly, hands on floor behind hips.

1 *Single Leg Extension:* Contract abdominals and round the spine. Bring knee toward chest, then extend leg straight ahead. Repeat 8 times; then change legs.

2 *Straight Leg Raise:* Same body position. Lock knee and tighten thigh muscles. Raise and lower straight leg 8 times.

3 *Progression:* Sit as erectly as possible, hands next to hip joints, and attempt to raise and lower straight leg again, this time without leaning back. This is challenging.

bike inner tubes

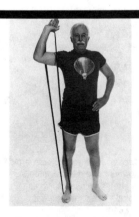 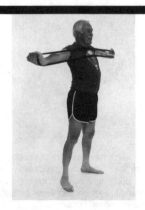

4 *Shoulder Flexibility:* Hook thumbs through tube and keep it taut. Touch thighs; then raise arms overhead and pull back. Bend elbows and touch tube to shoulder blades. Stretch tall again; then lower arms in front.

2 *Single Arm Push:* Stand on tube with right foot, right hand through tube, left hand on hip. Keeping body erect and legs straight, push up against tube, trying to bring hand to shoulder level. Repeat several times; then change to work with left arm. This exercise clearly demonstrates how much stronger the dominant arm is.

3 *Pectoral Toning:* Hold tube with arms at shoulder level, elbows slightly bent. Pull against tube to make it longer; then relax arms. Repeat five times. Do three sets.

4   **Side Leg Extension:** Lean back a little, hands behind you. Raise weighted straight leg just above floor, *toes pointing out*. Bring leg out to side as far as possible; then return to center, several times.

5   **Progression:** With legs straight and together, raise weighted leg a little, *toes pointing out*. Raise and lower leg, with foot turned out, to strengthen muscles on inside of thigh.

6   **Double Leg Raise:** Hold sand weight between feet. Lean back, supported by hands, and try to raise and lower straight legs without letting go of weight.

Lie down on your back to relax by shaking legs out, breathing deeply, and stretching tall.

Set #1: Upper Body Strength

1   **Garage Door Opener:** Stand on tube with feet about 1 ft apart. Place open palms under tube at chest level, hands shoulder-width apart. Bend knees, and push tube up as if opening a garage door while legs straighten. Try again, and push tube a little higher this time. Bike tubes are not very elastic, and individual arm strength will determine how much they will stretch. Inhale when knees bend; exhale when pushing against tube.

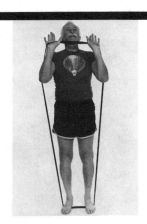

Cont.

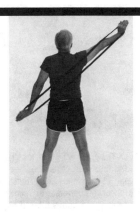

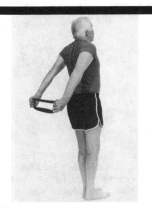

Many of the twisting, bending, and stretching movements suggested for dowels or webbing bands can be performed with folded inner tubes, adding a little elasticity to each movement. Use your imagination.

5   **Back Scratcher:** Keep tube behind back, and move it up and down along spine as if scratching your back.

6   **Posture Stretch:** Stand erect, folded tube held low behind hips. Pull arms away, stretching chest.

Set #2: Chair-Sitting Position

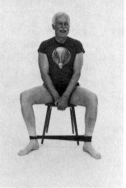

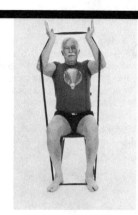

then pull out as far as possible, tensing muscles on outside of upper legs. Repeat slowly 10 times, keeping feet far enough apart.

2 Arm Strength: From same sitting position, step on open tube with feet hip-width apart. Place palms under tube at chest level. Push up to stretch tube, trying to bring hands to shoulder level. Inhale when relaxed; exhale when pushing.

1 Leg Strength: Sit tall, close to edge of chair. Place folded tube around ankles, and bring feet far enough apart to stretch tube tight. Let knees come toward each other;

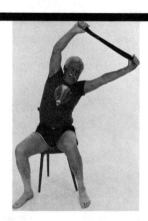

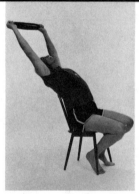

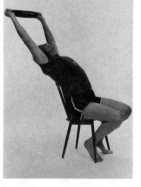

and inhale. Look up, and pull arms back more, arching lower back and stretching abdominal muscles. Lower arms and exhale.

5 Side Bending: With same leg position and arms overhead, hook thumbs through folded tube. Slowly bend right and left, keeping tube stretched.

6 Abdominal Stretch: Sit with feet together and lean back. Hook thumbs through folded tube, hands on thighs. Raise arms overhead

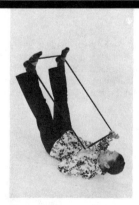

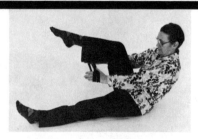

5 Sit-Up: A sit-up is made much easier by hanging onto this tube. Hold tube at chest level. Knees are bent, feet on tube. Lie down slowly, straightening legs, and keep head up. Sit up again as knees bend.

6 Leg Over Tube: Sit with legs together, and hold folded tube with arms stretched forward. Lean back a little. Bring right knee close to chest, and attempt to "climb" over tube, extending leg above tube. Bring knee to chest again to bring leg under tube and back to floor. Repeat with left leg and continue to alternate. This may be a little difficult for those with low back tightness and extra weight in the middle.

4 Back-Lying Square: Lie on your back to repeat this exercise with head and shoulders raised, legs up in the air. Really stretch tube to make the square as large as possible; then try to sit up. With good padding, this can turn into a rocking motion, sitting up and rolling back down again with legs in the air.

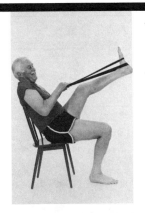

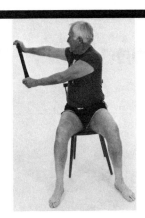

place foot on tube. Straighten leg forward; then pull it toward face, bending elbows. Try to keep knee straight. Hold for a few seconds and repeat with right leg.

4 **Upper Back Stretch:** Sit with legs far apart, feet firmly on floor. With arms forward at chest level, hook thumbs through folded tube. Looking at hands, pull tube slowly to the right, then to the left, upper body following arms.

3 **Leg Stretch:** Sit at edge of chair, upper back against chair back, double-folded tube held in both hands. Raise left knee and

Set #3: Floor-Sitting Position

Cont.

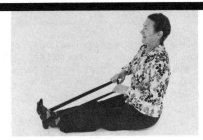

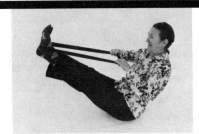

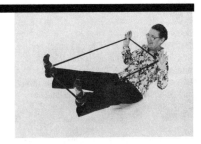

1 **Pectoral and Arm Strength:** Sit with legs together and straight, folded tube around feet. Grasp tube and pull it toward chest, bending elbows out and sitting tall.

2 **Balanced Leg Lift:** Sit with knees bent. Hold folded tube and place both feet on it. Lean back a little, and try to balance while legs straighten up at an angle for a V-sitting position. Balance by holding tube with both hands. The first attempt usually results in toppling over, so try several times.

3 **Square Tube:** Sit with feet hip-width apart on open tube, thumbs hooked through with hands shoulder-width apart. Raise legs and balance on buttocks. While balancing, push out with feet and pull with thumbs, shaping tube into a square.

Cont.

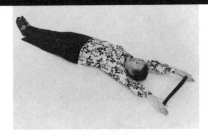

7 **Tall Stretch:** Lie on floor, arms overhead, open hands through folded tube, palms facing out. Push out, making tube taut, to stretch rib cage and waist, arms and shoulders, and to feel thin.

upholstery webbing bands

Set #1: Standing Stretches

1 **Straight Arm Twist:** With legs apart and arms forward at shoulder level, hold folded band taut. Instead of grasping band, push open hands through, palms facing out, to keep hands relaxed. Twist upper body slowly, keeping arms long and straight.

2 **Window Twist:** Hold folded band overhead. With legs well apart and head between arms, twist upper body and look through the "window" created by your arms.

3 **Twist and Bend:** With legs apart, hold arms overhead and band taut. Twist right and bend over right leg. Return to upright position, twist left, and bend over left leg.

Set #2: Stretching Shoulders, Chest, and Back of Body (Use folded band or inner tube.)

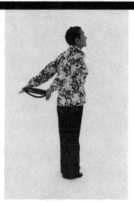 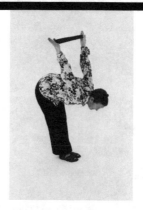 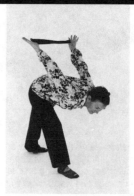

1 **Shoulder and Chest Stretch:** With legs together, stand erect, band held low behind hips. Without bending forward, pull straight arms away from back and look up. Hold for several seconds, relax arms, and repeat several more times.

2 **Hamstring and Back Stretch:** Stand with legs together, band held behind hips. Relax and bend forward, knees loose, and raise arms high behind you, bringing chest toward thighs. Straighten up slowly to avoid dizziness.

3 **Hamstring Stretch:** Take a small step forward at a slight angle with right leg, band held behind hips. Bend forward over straight right leg, bringing chest toward thigh, and pull arms up behind you. Hold for a few seconds, straighten up, and repeat, bending

4 *Continuous Circle:* With legs apart, hold arms overhead. Twist right, bend over right leg, continue along floor, and come up from the left. Circle several times, keeping knees loose; then change direction.

5 *Chest and Shoulder Stretch:* With legs together and arms overhead, hold band taut. Contract buttocks and abdominals. Pull straight arms back with easy bouncing movements. Lower arms to relax, and repeat once more.

over left leg. Repeat with band held overhead. Step forward with right leg, bend to touch band to foot, and hold to stretch. Stand erect again, arms overhead, and step forward with left leg.

Set #3: Sitting Stretches

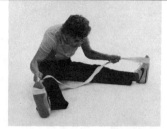

1 *Straight Leg Forward Bending:* Hold legs together and straight, one foot through each loop. Hold band near feet, bend forward at hip, and bring chest toward thighs. Pull upper body toward legs gently to stretch long back muscles, keeping chin up.

2 *Straddle Stretch:* Sit with legs apart, one foot through each loop. Hold band close to each foot, and bend forward between legs to bring chest toward floor. Keep chin up, back long and flat. Bounce chest lower with comfortable, easy movements, stretching low back muscles and insides of thighs.

3 *Alternate Leg Stretch:* With legs apart and one foot through each loop, turn upper body to face right leg. Hold band close to foot with both hands, and bend over right leg. Bring abdomen toward thigh, using band for anchoring. Hold this stretch, staying relaxed, before changing.

Set #4: Back-Lying Abdominals and Stretching

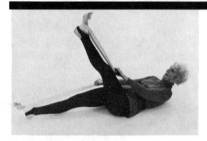

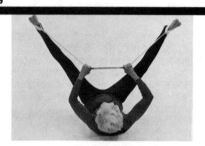

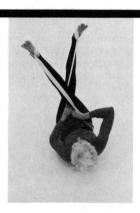

1 *Leg Scissoring:* Lie on back, feet through loops, head and shoulders up. Hold band near chest. Raise one straight leg high, keeping the other just above floor. Slowly move legs up and down in scissor pattern to strengthen abdominals. Focus on breathing rhythmically throughout and on locking lower back tightly to floor.

2 *Open/Cross Scissoring:* With head and shoulders up and legs high, hold band close to chest. Cross and open legs, toes pointing at ceiling. After a number of repetitions,

lower legs just a little to make the exercise more difficult. Keep lower back in contact with floor.

Set #5: Bands for Partner Stretching

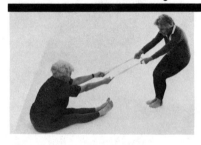

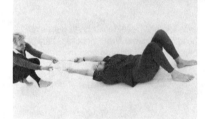

2 *Straddle Stretch:* Repeat with legs comfortably apart.

1 *Forward Stretching:* Partner A sits with legs straight and together, one hand through each loop. B stands in front of partner, holds band in both hands, and pulls A forward, arms and back long.

3 *Tall Stretch:* Lie on back, arms overhead, hands through loops. Partner stands several feet away from head and pulls against band, creating a long stretch in A's waistline, rib cage, and arms.

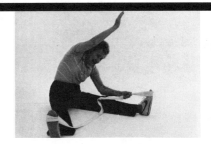

4 ___ *Side Bending:* Sit with legs apart, one foot through each loop, and hold band close to right foot with right hand. Raise left arm overhead, close to ear, and bend to reach toward right foot. Hold this stretch briefly, pulling against band; then sit erect and stretch to the left.

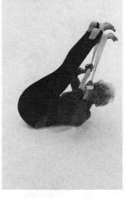

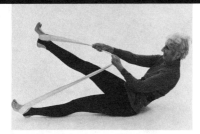

These bands are extremely helpful if low back and hamstring flexibility is poor. They help with anchoring for stability, resulting in better body positioning to stretch. When working with a partner, stretching becomes more effective still.

4 ___ *Tricky Sit-Up:* With legs straight on floor, hold band close to chest. Slowly curl upper body away from floor while right leg lifts. "Walk" hands along band toward right foot as you come up. From this V-sitting position, walk hands down while curling spine to floor and lowering leg. Repeat with left leg.

3 ___ *Double Leg and Hip Stretch:* Raise both legs; lift head and shoulders. Pull legs toward face, raising hips away from floor. Good padding for spine is important.

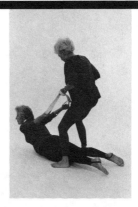

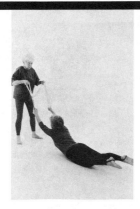

4 ___ *Posture Stretch:* Roll over onto stomach, arms along body, hands still through loops. B stands, straddling A's lower legs, and pulls as A raises chest and chin away from floor and brings arms back.

5 ___ *Variation:* B stands in front of A, whose arms are held in a wide V position. B pulls partner's arms and chest up from floor and holds for a few seconds to stretch. Lower slowly.

scarves

Waving and Swinging, for graceful and energetic movements. Each person has two scarves.

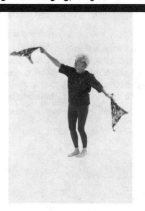

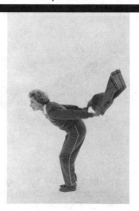

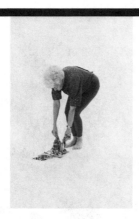

1 *Scissor Arm Swing:* Stand with legs together. Swing one arm forward, the other back, with light, rhythmical knee bending.

2 *Double Arm Swing:* Both arms swing forward, then way back, with more vigorous knee bending.

3 *Touch and Stretch:* With legs together, bend knees and touch scarves to floor. Straighten legs, stretch arms into a wide V, and look up.

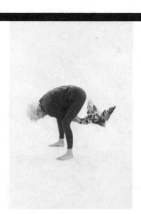

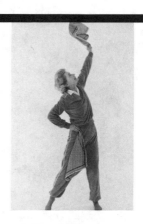

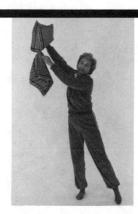

7 *Swing and Stretch:* With legs apart, bend forward to swing scarves through legs; then straighten up and stretch arms into a wide V.

8 *Single Arm Fling:* Legs apart and right hand on hip, swing left arm over right shoulder, then out at left. Repeat several times with each arm, and push off with feet.

9 *Double Arm Swing:* Repeat movement, swinging both arms over right and left shoulder while weight shifts from one foot to the other.

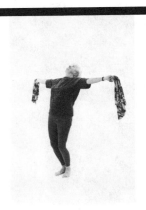

4 *Single Arm Circling:* With legs together, alternately circle arms from front to back, completing each circle before other arm moves.

5 *Backward Windmill:* Speed up this movement for continuous, energetic windmilling from front to back.

6 *Forward Windmill:* With legs apart, windmill arms forward with energetic movements.

Cont.

10 *Flying:* Extend arms at shoulder level. Turn them into wings with an up-and-down flying motion.

11 *Arm Crossing:* Stand with legs together. While knees bend and straighten, cross and open arms.

12 *Crossover Arm Circling:* Cross arms in front, and circle up and around to cross overhead again. Bend knees when arms cross low, rise up on toes when arms cross overhead.

13 *Combination:* Cross and open arms. Then cross to circle up and around while bending knees lightly.

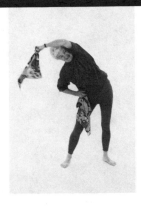

14 *Waving:* Stand with legs apart, one hand on hip, other arm overhead. Wave with large arm movement, bending right and left. Think of a palm tree swaying in the breeze.

15 *Double Arm Circling:* With legs apart, swing scarves in large circles from the right along floor to left and high overhead, keeping arms close together. Circle several times each way.

16 *Dust Shaker:* Stand with arms forward at shoulder level. Moving wrists vigorously, shake scarves while holding arms straight and moving out and forward again.

Cont.

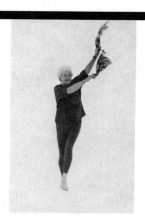

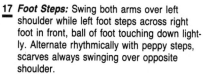

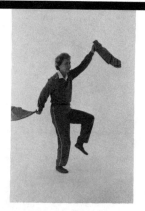

Scarves for swinging and waving add color and variety to many of the walking, skipping, and waltzing patterns. Scarves bring lightness to the variety of steps and help with coordination. Waltzing with scarves looks especially graceful, and it's uplifting on a dreary day. Coordinating various arm swinging patterns while standing in circle formation can make even a beginning class look great. Again, experiment with your own ideas and add more activities to those suggested here.

17 ***Foot Steps:*** Swing both arms over left shoulder while left foot steps across right foot in front, ball of foot touching down lightly. Alternate rhythmically with peppy steps, scarves always swinging over opposite shoulder.

18 ***Hop and Swing:*** Swing scarves forward and back while hopping from one foot on the other, pulling knee up.

6
floor
exercises

Many seniors programs do not include floor exercises, instead relying on chairs for safe positioning. Many older people have real fears about lowering themselves to the floor and getting stuck there, not knowing how to get up again safely. For many, it's hard enough to get out of a soft chair once comfortably settled, and without careful step-by-step practice, getting down onto the floor is truly not safe. This is a good example of having lost the body confidence to do something that used to be easy, simply because it is no longer part of everyday living. As children and young people, we often spend more time on the floor than in chairs. But as we get to be middle-aged, this no longer seems appropriate, and we conform. Hunkering is comfortable for people in many cultures, and elders sit cross-legged for their council meetings. It's societal conditioning that makes our bodies more or less comfortable with different ways of sitting, and if you have been to a Japanese tea house, you know that eating at floor level can be a miserable experience if you seldom spend time this way.

Young people are agile enough to complete a sequence of movements like sitting down and getting up from the floor without thinking. But when muscles are weak and joints stiff, this movement sequence becomes a matter of safety and has to be thought about and practiced. We go through the following drill regularly, and as a result everyone in our group feels safe and comfortable getting down onto the floor for many of the exercises.

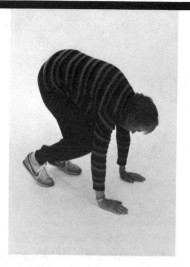
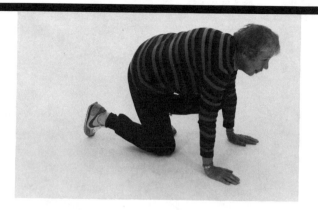

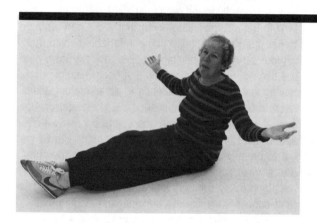

I demonstrate slowly, step by step, and then we practice together:

1. Bend your knees enough to place hands solidly on floor.
2. Lower one knee to the floor so that you have a tripod support.
3. Lower other knee to floor to be on all fours now.
4. Sit on one buttock, hands still in contact with floor for stability.
5. Straighten legs out in front of you now, and you're safely seated.

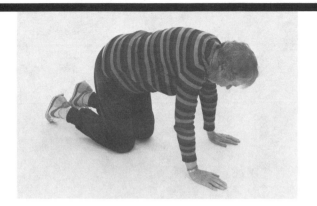

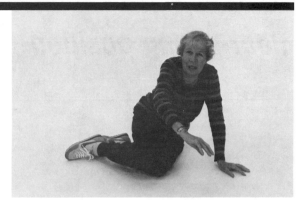

Cont.

To get up, simply reverse the process:

1. Bend knees, bring them to one side, and sit on that buttock. Place both hands firmly on floor next to hip.
2. Get onto all fours.
3. Raise one knee and put foot on floor.
4. Raise hips and other knee. Both feet and hands are in solid contact with floor while in this squatting position.
5. Use thigh muscles to straighten up.

This practice and development of body confidence has resulted in total loss of fear for my students. Some had given up relaxing baths, showering instead, because they were too afraid of lowering themselves into the tub and struggling to get out again. Body confidence allows a soothing bath to remain a special, relaxing treat at the end of the day, eliminating the need for holding on to faucets or soap dishes as some had done before. And many of my students often sit on the floor at home now, just for fun.

floor-sitting position

Set #1: Upper Body Strengthening

<u>1</u>   ***Bent-Knee Body Lift:*** Sit with knees bent, feet on floor, hip-width apart, and hands on floor behind hips. Push up to raise hips high, hold briefly, and sit down.

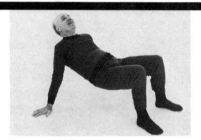

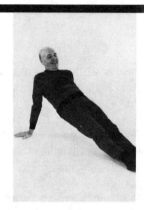

<u>2</u>   ***Straight Leg Body Lift:*** Sit with legs together and straight. Lean back, hands behind hips. Raise body to bring it into a straight line, and inhale. Return hips to floor and exhale.

Set #2: Hip Joint Limbering

<u>1</u>   ***Knee Drops:*** Sit with knees bent, feet together, hands behind hips. Push knees to the right until right leg touches down. Roll across hips and bring knees to the left. Look at raised hip to twist and limber the lower back.

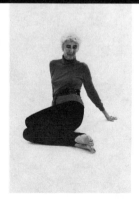

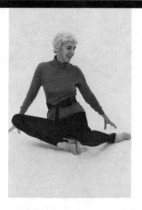

<u>2</u>   ***Open Knee Drop:*** Repeat this movement with feet and knees hip-width apart, touching both legs to floor each time. Look at raised buttock.

3 *Progression #1:* Sit very straight, palms firmly placed next to hips. Raise hips just a few inches away from floor; lower them carefully.

4 *Progression #2:* This requires good wrist strength. Sit, leaning back again, hands behind you. Keep legs straight and together. Raise body up into a straight line, and then try to lift one leg just a little. Sit down to relax; then repeat, lifting other leg.

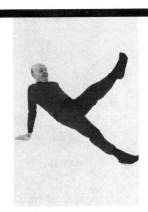

5 Relax by bending forward over relaxed legs, upper body and arms loose.

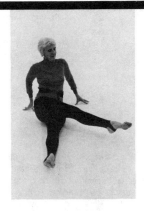

3 *Crossover Leg Swing:* Leaning back, hands behind you, sit with legs straight. Lift right leg, and swing it across the left leg, big toe touching floor. In an arc, swing leg far out to the right, little toe touching down.

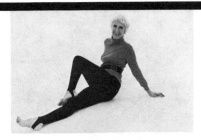

4 *Knee Crossover:* Sit with hands behind you. Keep right leg straight, and place left foot on right knee. Push knee across toward floor at right with gentle bouncing movements to stretch out hip joint and outside of hip. Repeat with other knee.

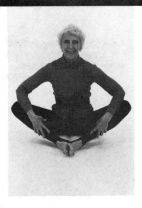

5 *Butterfly:* Sit tall, soles of feet together, knees pointing out. Hold ankles from inside and place elbows against knees. Gently push knees out with small bouncing movements to limber hip joints. Then bend forward between open knees, back round and relaxed.

Set #3: Back and Leg Stretching

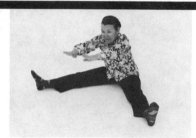

1 **Forward Bending:** Extend arms forward, chin up, legs apart. Bend forward and reach with one arm at a time as if hauling in a fishing line.

2 **Breast Stroke:** With legs apart, swim the breast stroke, bending forward with long arms, then opening arms wide to stretch chest in erect sitting position.

Set #4: Leg Stretching

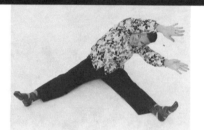 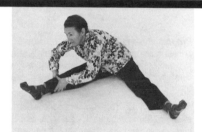

1 **Stretch and Bend:** Sit tall, legs straight and together, arms high, and inhale. Bend forward at hip, and bring abdomen toward thighs. Try to touch toes, arms and back long, and exhale.

2 **Alternate Leg Stretch:** With legs apart, arms high, inhale. Bend over right leg, touch hands to foot, and exhale. Sit up again, reach tall, and bend over left leg.

3 **Sustained Leg Stretch:** Legs apart, turn to face right leg. Bend over leg and place hands under calf. Gently pull chest toward leg with very gentle, small pulsing movements. Chin is up, back flat, and knee relaxed. Repeat, bending over left leg.

Set #5: Back and Leg Stretching

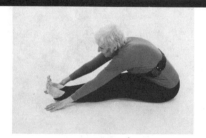 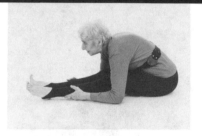

1 **Forward Stretch:** Sit with legs straight and together, arms extended forward at shoulder level, chin up. Reach forward with one arm at a time, pulling an imaginary rope toward you.

2 **Finger Walk:** Legs together, hands on floor, walk fingers toward feet. Hold the longest stretch for a few seconds, and walk back.

3 **Sustained Stretch:** With legs together, place palms under calves and keep knees slightly bent. Bring upper body toward legs by bending elbows out rather than pulling chest down. Bounce gently and loosely, keeping back straight.

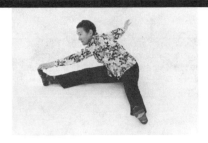 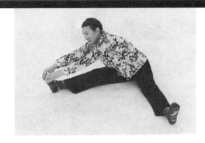

3 *Alternate Toe Touch:* With legs apart, extend arms out at shoulder level. Bend forward and reach across to touch right hand to left foot, left hand to right foot.

4 *Foot to Foot Swing:* With legs apart, bring both hands to right foot, then to left foot, upper body following arm movement. Relax hamstring muscles by shaking legs.

4 *Finger Walk:* Legs apart, turn to face right leg, hands on floor at either side of knee. Slowly walk fingertips toward foot and bring chest closer to thigh. Hold the longest stretch for several seconds, return to upright position, and walk fingers along left leg.

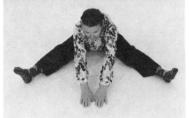

6 Bend knees to relax hamstring muscles.

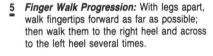

5 *Finger Walk Progression:* With legs apart, walk fingertips forward as far as possible; then walk them to the right heel and across to the left heel several times.

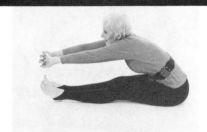 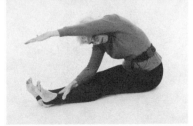

6 *Body Lift:* Hands behind hips, raise body into a straight line, weight on heels and hands only, to stretch shoulders, chest, and abdominals.

4 *Pushaway:* Keep legs together and hold hands. Bend forward and push palms forward at shoulder level, stretching fingers, arms, back, and legs.

5 *Crossover Stretch:* With legs together and knees relaxed, grasp left lower leg with right hand. Bring left arm up from behind in a high arc and try to touch fingers to floor next to right ankle. Return arm in a high arc and change.

Set #6: Upper Back and Neck Stretching

1 *Upper Back Stretch:* Legs together and hands on shoulders, bend forward with rounded back and bring elbows toward knees. Then sit tall and push elbows back to stretch chest.

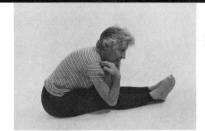

2 *Upper Back and Neck Stretch:* With legs together, lace hands behind neck. Again, bend forward with rounded upper back and slowly bring elbows toward knees. This is a strong stretch; don't attempt to touch legs.

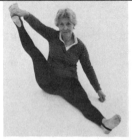

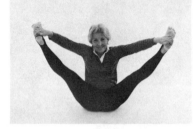

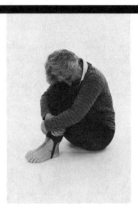

5 *Balance Challenge:* Sit with soles of feet touching, knees out. Right hand holds right heel from *inside*; left hand is on floor for support. Attempt to straighten right leg up at an angle. Return foot to floor and stretch left leg.

6 *Balance Challenge With Both Legs:* Now hold both heels with both hands and try to stretch both legs into a wide V. There will be little success on the first few attempts, and loss of balance will cause general tumbling back. Abdominals have to be contracted to help with balance.

7 *Cuddle Up:* Bend knees, feet on floor. Wrap arms around lower legs and bring forehead to knees.

3 *Elbow to Floor:* Legs apart and hands on shoulders. Bend to the right and try to touch elbow to floor. Sit up, then touch left elbow down. Stabilize body by keeping legs well apart.

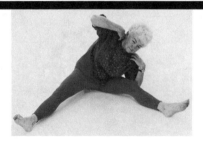

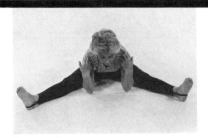 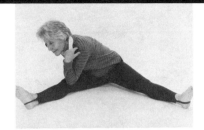

3 *Elbows to Floor:* With legs apart, put hands on shoulders. Bend forward, back rounded, and touch elbows to floor. Come into an erect sitting position, and push elbows back to stretch chest.

4 *Elbow to Knee:* With legs apart and hands on shoulders, turn to the left and bring right elbow toward left knee. Sit upright; then bring left elbow toward right knee.

Set #7: Waistline Stretching

Cont.

1 *Raised Arm Stretch:* Sit with legs apart, left hand holding left ankle. Raise right arm straight up and bend toward left leg. Hold for a few seconds, arm stretching long, and change slowly.

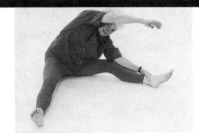

2 *Trunk Circling:* Legs apart, hook thumbs together overhead. Circle arms and upper body to the right; reach far over, bring hands along floor to the left, and come up and around several times. Change direction.

Cont.

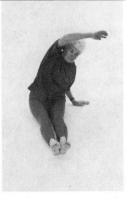

5 *Rib Cage Lifting:* With legs together, interlace fingers and raise arms overhead. Stretch arms and rib cage, palms facing ceiling. Really push up to feel a strong stretch. Exhale and lower arms.

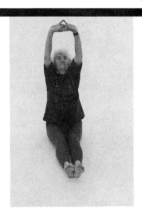

4 *Tall Side Bending:* Legs together, put left hand on floor near hip. Lift right arm straight up, and keep it close to ear while bending to the left. Hold and bounce gently; then change.

Set #8: Twist, Bend, and Stretch

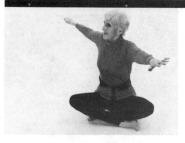 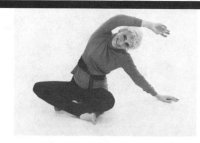 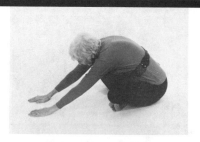

1 *Trunk Twisting:* Sit with legs crossed, spine straight. Extend arms out at shoulder level. Twist upper body right and left, following movement with eyes.

2 *Side Bending:* With legs crossed, keep left hand on floor in line with hip joint. Bring right arm overhead, and bend to the left without raising buttock. Alternate several times, stretching slowly.

3 *Spine Stretching:* With legs crossed, reach forward with both arms and touch hands to floor, arms long. Sit up and open arms wide at shoulder level.

abdominal exercises

As long as older persons are still pursuing an active, independent lifestyle that includes walking, doing their own house and yard work, and climbing stairs, most retain a reasonable level of overall muscular strength. But when I ask my students which area they feel needs improvement most, all hands automatically pat the midsection: Abdominal muscles are weak, and fat has settled in this area; it seems hardest to make changes there. Over the years, men's midsections have a tendency to "go to pot," and many women develop protruding abdomens and "spare tires." These physical changes are very typical of aging, along with such postural changes as a rounded upper back, unless people have stayed physically very active throughout life.

For women, especially, a strong abdominal girdle provides the necessary support for internal organs. If muscles are not kept strong through midlife, they will no longer give this support. Much like a worn-out elastic girdle, abdominals stretch and become too long and weak. This, combined with the natural forces of gravity, allows internal organs to push against the abdominal wall, stretching muscles and resulting in the protruding lower abdomen so very common in older women, even those who are thin. Well-directed exercise can certainly give these muscles better tone, but the basic shape of an older body is not likely to change with sit-ups. Fat can be lost and clothes will fit better, but the thickened waistline is truly one of the characteristics of older age, unless a person has remained thin and fit throughout

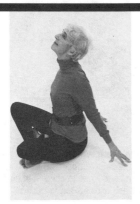

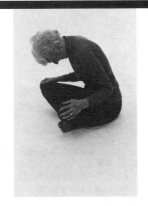

5 *Trunk Circling:* Combine some of these movements into a pattern: Bend right, left arm overhead. Next, bring arms and upper body forward to stretch far ahead. Bend left, right arm overhead. Now place hands behind hips, straighten spine, and push shoulders back and chin up. Repeat slowly three times; then change direction for three more circles.

4 *Chest and Shoulder Stretch:* With legs crossed, sit tall, palms behind hips. Look up and push shoulders back. Inhale. Relax upper body and arms, slumping forward, and exhale. Repeat several times.

life. We have to help participants be realistic about the cosmetic effects of exercise. Certain bodily changes are a normal part of the aging process and must be accepted. At 70, we cannot regain the youthful shape of a 20-year-old, and it is important not to make such promises. But we can work at *looking our very best for our age*, and that is a very realistic goal. The most noticeable improvement possible is postural, the way we carry ourselves. An older person can impress through a youthful carriage, and appropriate clothing can hide some of the figure faults.

Abdominal exercises are important for a number of reasons. They help restore muscle tone, even though it may not be outwardly visible. As does improved posture, stronger abdominals help protect the lower back. Abdominal exercises also play an important role in improved digestion, massaging the intestinal tract and helping food move along more efficiently. Many older people rely on laxatives, but they can be encouraged to replace these with regular daily abdominal exercises, and by eating enough foods with fiber and drinking more fluids.

As participants get ready for abdominal exercises, there is often general groaning because these muscles are so weak. The exercises have to be portioned out in small doses, always alternating with relaxing exercises after a short set. As mentioned, there is no good reason for a high number of repetitions of any exercise. As soon as abdominal muscles become fatigued, there is a

tendency for the pelvis to push forward and the lower back to arch. Continuing will be a struggle, often resulting in an aching lower back instead of stronger abdominals. Use good judgment and let the class guide you. With a new class, start with easy exercises and progress slowly to avoid discouraging your students and stressing their lower backs. Remind everyone of good breathing, inhaling when relaxed and exhaling when muscles contract. Oxygen has to keep coming in to fuel working muscles. Talk about good breathing while exercising to help students combat the tendency to hold their breath on the more demanding exercises. Remember, too, that rhythmical breathing is especially important for those with high blood pressure.

Set #1: Back-Lying Abdominals

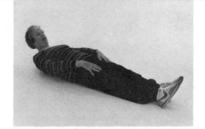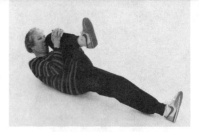

1 *Low Back Press:* Lie down on mat, knees bent, feet on floor, arms relaxed along body. Arch lower back slightly and inhale. Then contract abdominal muscles, press lower back tightly to floor, and hold for a few seconds while exhaling.

2 *Head and Shoulder Lift:* With legs straight and hands on thighs, inhale. Raise head and shoulders, fingertips reaching for knees, and exhale while looking at feet.

3 *Knee to Chest:* With legs together and straight, inhale. Lift head and shoulders, pull one knee close to chest with both hands, and exhale. Return to floor, inhale, and pull other knee up.

Set #2: Back-Lying Abdominals

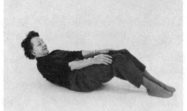

1 *Quarter Sit-Up:* Keep knees bent, feet on floor, arms overhead. Raise head and upper back while hands reach forward to touch knees. Bounce forward several times, keeping lower back pressed to floor. Relax, stretching arms overhead and inhaling deeply.

2 *Elbow to Knee:* With hands on shoulders and legs straight, raise upper body and right leg, twisting to touch left elbow to outside of right knee. Return to floor. Repeat, raising left leg.

Set #3: Back-Lying Abdominals

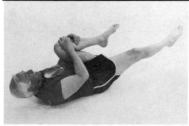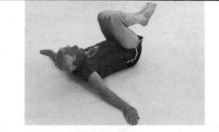

2 *Single Leg Pump:* Keep one knee close to chest, head up. Other leg is long and straight. Raise and lower this leg slowly 10 times. Change.

1 *Single Leg Extension:* Start with head and shoulders up, one knee pulled close to chest, hands around knee. The other leg is very straight and held just above floor. Alternate rhythmically, pulling one knee close while other leg extends. Focus on good breathing.

3 *Double Leg Extension:* Extend arms out at shoulder level. Bring both knees to chest; then extend legs straight up. Again, bend knees into chest, and extend legs a little lower this time, lifting head and shoulders to keep back from arching. Inhale on bending; exhale on extending legs.

4 ***Single Leg Raise:*** With legs straight and arms overhead, inhale. Raise arms, head, upper back and right leg, and try to touch hands to right foot while exhaling. Slowly return to floor. Repeat, raising left leg.

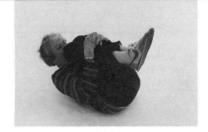

5 ***Double Knee to Chest:*** Inhale. Lift head and shoulders, bring both knees to chest, and wrap arms around lower legs while exhaling. Relax, stretching arms and legs for a deep breath, and curl up again.

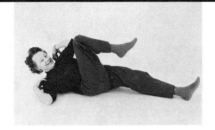

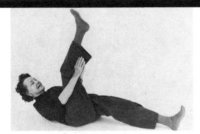

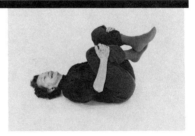

3 ***Elbow to Bent Knee:*** In same position, put hands on shoulders. Raise upper back while bringing right knee toward chest and twist to touch left elbow to knee. Return to floor, inhale, and touch right elbow to left knee.

4 ***Handclap Leg Raise:*** Extend arms out at shoulder level. Raise upper back and straight right leg, and clap hands behind knee. Return to floor, inhale, and raise left leg.

5 Relax by crossing ankles and pulling knees toward outsides of chest, hands around knees, to stretch lower back.

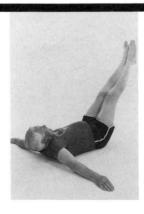

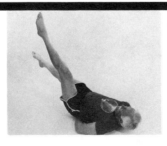

5 Relax by stretching tall, arms overhead, as you inhale deeply. Curl into a tight ball and exhale.

4 ***Scissor Kick:*** With head and shoulders up and hands under buttocks, raise right leg high, and slowly lower it halfway while left leg comes up. Continue scissoring your legs as you breathe rhythmically. Keep lower back in contact with floor throughout.

Set #4: Floor-Sitting Abdominals

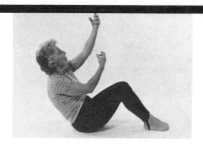

1 *Curl-Down:* With knees bent and hands on knees, tuck chin close to chest, spine rounded, and inhale. Slide hands along thighs, slowly curling spine to floor while exhaling. Keep abdominals contracted. Return to sitting position using hands to push up from floor, and repeat.

2 *Half Curl-Down:* Same sitting position, back rounded, and chin close to chest. Curl down just halfway; then try to return to sitting position, keeping hands on thighs. Even the attempt is good exercise.

3 *Lifeline:* Sit with knees bent, arms raised. Pretend there is a rope: With hand-over-hand movement, slowly lower spine to floor with the help of this imaginary lifeline. Try to come up, hanging on to the rope, one hand reaching above the other. This is a struggle, especially on coming up.

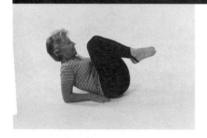

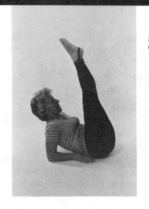

6 Relax with tall stretching, lying down, then shaking legs out.

5 *Double Leg Extension:* In same half-sitting position, bring both knees to chest and extend legs up. Bring knees to chest again, then return feet to floor, touching down

lightly and forward enough to feel abdominals contract. The pattern is bend, stretch, bend, touch down.

2 *Legs Apart/Together:* In same sitting position, lean back a little so that legs can move freely. Raise legs enough to bring them apart, heels touching floor. Raise legs again to return to starting position.

3 *Combination:* Combine these last two movements: Bend knees, extend legs forward on floor, bring legs apart and back together.

4 *Bicycle:* Lean back on lower arms for a bicycling motion with both legs. Stretch each leg long as it extends forward.

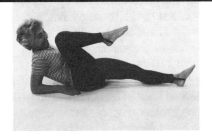 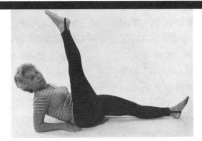

4 *Single Leg Extension:* In half-sitting position, place hands far behind hips and bring lower arms to floor for good upper body support. Contract abdominals and press lower back to floor. Bring one knee toward nose, extend leg straight up, and lower it to floor. Repeat several times with same leg before changing.

Set #5: Floor-Sitting Abdominals

Cont.

1 *Rowing:* Keep legs straight, hands on floor near hips. Lean back enough to touch lower arms to floor, keeping spine round. Sit up, bending knees and touching nose to knees.

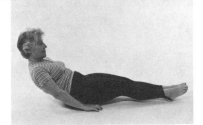 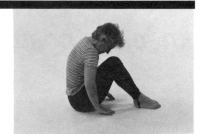

Cont.

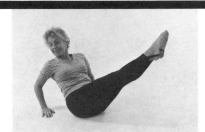 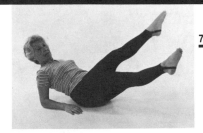

7 Relax on back, knees bent, feet on floor, arms along body. Slowly raise tailbone and rest of spine to stretch abdominal muscles and chest while inhaling. Curl spine back to floor slowly, exhaling.

5 *Side Leg Extension:* Lean back a little, hands on floor, knees close to chest. Roll across hips to the right, and extend both legs to the right just above floor. Bend knees, roll across hips to the left, and extend legs to the left.

6 *Sitting Scissor:* Lean back, supported by lower arms, and raise legs 2 ft above floor. Open and cross legs rhythmically, but keep legs high enough to prevent back arching. Focus on good breathing. Pull abdominals in strongly to keep lower back rounded.

A major complaint often arises during abdominal exercises: the discomfort of neck muscles tensing and tiring from repeated head and shoulder lifting. In order to perform abdominal exercises safely and correctly, the spine must always be rounded so that the lower back maintains contact with the floor instead of arching away. This happens as soon as head and shoulders are raised, making this body positioning necessary, especially for those with poor abdominal strength. So we are confronted by a predicament because the neck discomfort is a recurring problem and hard to prevent. Since these important exercises should not be eliminated, make sure not to do too many at one time in the back-lying position where head and shoulder raising is necessary. One set of chair-sitting abdominals can be combined with one set of floor exercises and followed with relaxing movements for the neck, or with self-massage.

Another solution is to do one set of abdominals early on in the class, and come back to these muscles again toward the end, just before spending time with stretching and relaxing. In addition, encourage your students to do simple abdominal contractions at home whenever they think of it: Either standing or sitting, pull abdominal muscles in very hard for a few seconds, relax, and repeat several times. This is easy to do while standing in line at the bank or grocery store checkout, while driving or watching television. If buttocks are contracted at the same time, both muscle groups get needed exercise. It's these few minutes spent daily that can make a big difference.

Another negative experience for some is dizziness when lying flat. Instead of not participating in floor exercises, those with this problem should bring a small pillow to class. If the problem persists, chair-sitting abdominals can be substituted.

kneeling position

The kneeling position may be uncomfortable for some. There are those with arthritic knees, knee injuries, and even knee replacements who are concerned about the pressure created by placing weight on the knees. Good padding is a must, and some may have to use two or three carpet squares to be comfortable. Encourage everyone to participate in these exercises unless it really creates problems. This may be the only reasonable position in which an older person can continue gardening, for example. Knee pads can be purchased or made for yard and housework, and that is preferable to giving up these activities. Unless a person has a physician's direction not to kneel, push a little for participation, again explaining the importance for daily living.

This raises the interesting question of where discomfort ends and pain starts, something which is difficult to judge. Each one of us has a different pain threshold and a different level of toughness. Basically, exercise should not cause pain unless a diagnosed condition exists which precludes pain-free movement. Pain that has no explanation should be diagnosed, and medical advice regarding exercise be given. What may register as discomfort in some may be experienced as a very real pain by others. We should rely on the individual's good judgment and common sense in this respect. Arthritic flare-ups, tendon inflammation, or bursitis can present a rainbow of pain levels, and a physician's advice should be heeded. In general, adhere to the "use it or lose it" principle, but exercise certainly needs to be adjusted to work around an existing problem. Rely on medical advice shared with the individual, and beyond that on the person's good decision making. Even if a number of exercises need to be eliminated, there is still a lot to be gained from participation in general. A person recovering from a broken wrist obviously cannot and should not do push-ups, for example, but the rest of the body is in need of movement and should not be put to rest because of a wrist injury.

Set #1: Low Back Limbering, Buttock Strengthening

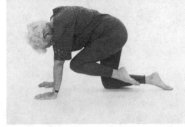

1 *Cat Back:* On all fours, contract abdominals and round the spine like an angry cat. Relax, arching the back a little while looking up. Repeat slowly several times, with focus on strong abdominal contractions. Continue more rapidly for low back limbering.

3 *Angle Knee to Shoulder:* Change the angle of this leg movement by bringing knee toward opposite shoulder, then extending leg catty-cornered behind you.

2 *Knee to Nose:* Bring one knee toward nose, rounding spine. Then extend leg behind you to contract buttock muscles. Repeat several times; then change.

Set #2: Low Back Limbering, Buttock Strengthening

1 *Straight Leg Raise:* Extend one leg behind you, toes pointed. Raise and lower straight leg 10 times without arching lower back.

2 *Side Leg Raise:* Extend one leg out to side. With good support from hands and other knee, raise and lower leg in this position.

3 *Arc Leg Lift:* From this position, raise leg and bring it behind you in an arc, big toe touching down. Lift again and return leg to side. A few repetitions will be enough.

Set #3: Limbering and Stretching

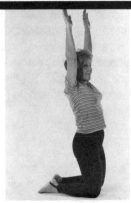 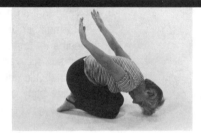 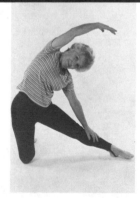

1 *Stretch and Curl:* Kneeling with arms overhead, stretch tall. Now swing arms down and behind you while bending at the hip and rounding the spine. Head comes toward knees. Return to upright position and repeat several times, exhaling forcefully when bending.

2 *Side Bending:* Kneel upright. Extend left leg out, foot on floor. Place left hand on left leg and raise right arm straight up. Bend to the left, and let hand slide along leg toward ankle. Keep right arm straight and close to ear. Slowly return to upright position. Repeat several times before changing.

4 *Leg Circling:* Extend one leg straight back, toes pointed. Raise it to hip level and draw circles from outside in. Change legs.

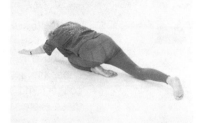

5 *Leg and Back Stretch:* Stretch left leg far back, foot on floor, while hips move back to touch right heel and arms stretch forward, hands on floor. Hold this stretch for a few seconds; then raise hips and bring knee forward. Repeat, stretching other leg far back.

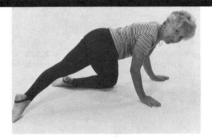

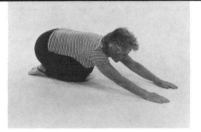

4 *Low Leg Crossover:* Same starting position, keep foot on floor now. Draw a half circle along floor with big toe, crossing leg over behind you. Look over opposite shoulder as leg crosses over, creating a twisting motion at the waist. Bend elbows as leg swings behind you. Repeat several times with same leg to stretch outside of hip and hip joint.

5 Relax by sitting back on heels, arms and back stretched long. Inch forward with one hand at a time without raising hips.

3 *Palms Up Stretch:* Kneel upright. Hold hands overhead, fingers laced, and palms facing up. Stretch very tall, pushing palms higher. Look up and inhale deeply. Separate hands and lower arms, reaching out while exhaling. Repeat several times.

4 *Hip Wagging:* On all fours, knees hip-width apart, push hips from side to side to limber lower back. Combine slow and fast hip swinging.

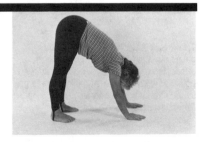

5 *Triangle Stretch:* From all-fours position, raise hips high to bring weight onto feet and hands, body in a triangle. Push heels toward floor, and work at stretching out all muscles in back of body. Stay in this triangle position for a slow count of 10; then bend knees to return to floor.

front-lying position

Exercises performed in a front-lying position contract and strengthen muscles in the back of the body. Raising arms or trunk strengthens shoulders, upper arms, and upper back. Various leg-raising movements contract and strengthen buttock muscles. Follow sets of these exercises with low back stretching, and use good padding to protect pelvic bones and ribs from the hard floor.

Keeping buttock muscles strong is as important as maintaining good abdominal muscle tone. These two major muscle groups should provide strong support for the lower spine and act as a natural girdle. Good posture, too, depends on these important muscles, bringing the pelvis into good alignment and minimizing the likelihood or degree of swayback.

Set #1: Upper Back, Shoulder Girdle, and Upper Arm Strengthening

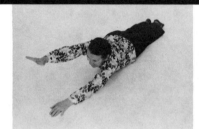

1 *Single Arm Raise:* Extend arms forward. Raise and lower one arm at a time, keeping head low.

2 *Single Arm Arc:* Extend arms forward. Raise head, and lift one arm in an arc to rest along lower body. Return arm forward and repeat this movement several times. Repeat with other arm.

Set #2: Back, Shoulders, Upper Arms

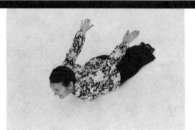
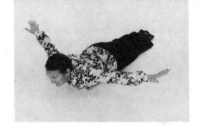

1 *Trunk Raising:* With arms along body, palms up, slowly raise chin, chest, and arms. Return to floor slowly. This is a controlled *lifting* motion to strengthen the large supporting back muscles along the spine. Do not swing up! Don't raise trunk any higher than is comfortable.

2 *Progression:* Extend arms at shoulder level, palms down. Raise and lower trunk slowly several times. Back muscles contract adequately if trunk is raised slightly; there should be little low back arching.

3 *Arm Circling:* Extend arms at shoulder level, palms down. Raise chin and chest a little while arms describe small circles, moving from front to back.

4 *Upper Arm Toner:* With chin on floor and arms along body, turn palms up. Push arms toward ceiling with small bouncing movements, keeping them straight and close to body.

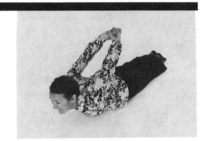

5 *Chest and Shoulder Stretch:* Hold hands behind back. Pull straight arms away from body, hold for a few seconds, relax, and repeat again.

3 *Progression:* Chin on hands. Lift chin, arms, and chest slowly and with control, just high enough to feel back muscles contract. Slowly return to floor.

4 Relax and stretch lower back after these movements by coming up onto all fours. Push hips back, close to heels, for a long back stretch.

Set #3: Push-Up Series

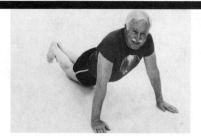 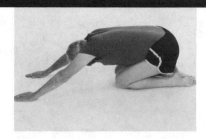

1 *Easy Push-Away:* Place palms near shoulders. Slowly push away from floor, straightening arms and looking up. Contract buttock muscles to prevent low back arching. Slowly return to floor.

2 *Push-Up/Back Stretch:* Push up as above; then push hips back to touch heels, stretching arms and back long. Raise hips, shift weight forward onto hands, bend elbows, and return to floor.

Set #4: Low Back/Buttock Strengthening

1 *Single Leg Raise:* Chin on hands, raise straight right leg to feel buttock muscles contract. Push leg toward ceiling with bouncing movements; then change legs.

2 *Single Leg Out/In:* Chin on right hand, extend left arm at an angle for balance. Lift right leg out, touch foot to floor, and return leg to center. Repeat several times with each leg.

3 *Buttock Firmer:* Chin on hands, bring legs apart and touch feet to floor; then bring legs together again. Try to raise legs completely away from floor for each movement.

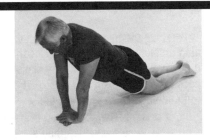
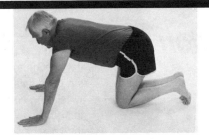
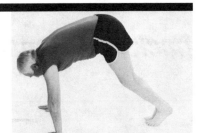

3   *Hand-on-Hand Push-Up:* This is a more difficult push-up version. Rest on lower arms, one hand covering the other at chest level. Slowly straighten arms, pushing against floor with heels of hands to bring upper body away from floor. Legs stay down.

4   *Triangle Push-Up:* On all fours, toes curled under, raise hips high and straighten legs to come into a triangle position. Push heels toward floor to stretch lower legs, and hold for a few seconds. Bend knees to kneel again.

4   *Leg Circling:* Chin on right hand, extend left arm at an angle for balance. Raise right leg, and draw circles through the air, moving outward. Change legs.

5   *Buttock Contraction:* Chin on hands, contract buttocks as tightly as possible and hold for several seconds. Relax, and let heels turn out. Repeat several times.

6   Relax with a long body stretch: Arms extended forward, inch forward with one hand at a time, pushing away with feet at the same time.

Many of these exercises are not easy, so just a short set should be done in each class. The front-lying position may not be comfortable for some, and those who are thin need to use two carpet squares to protect pelvic bones. If some participants choose to sit out these exercises, be supportive of their decision. Working with light weights in a standing position strengthens these muscles, too, and can be a substitute. Respect the individual's decision to do what feels right and comfortable. There is more to be gained from eliminating some exercises than miserably struggling through them.

back-lying position

Some persons experience dizziness when lying flat. Suggest that they bring a small pillow to raise the head just enough to avoid this problem. The end of the class is a good time for these back-lying exercises, followed by relaxing and deep breathing. This is an enjoyable and quieting way to end a class. I have separated the abdominal exercises from these sets because they spell hard work and are not appropriate for the end of the hour.

Set #1: Hip and Body Raising

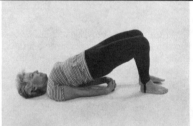

1 *Buttock Lift:* Knees bent, feet hip-width apart, arms along body, raise hips to knee level, contracting buttocks strongly. Feel thigh muscles work, too. Lower hips to floor, and repeat until buttock muscles feel tired.

2 *Spine Lifting:* In same starting position, contract abdominals and press lower back tightly to floor. Starting with tailbone, slowly curl spine away from floor. Feel each vertebra come up separately. Come up to shoulder blades, inhaling deeply. Then curl spine down slowly, one vertebra at a time, exhaling. This exercise works on abdominal control, spinal flexibility, and stretching front of body.

3 *Spine Lifting With Stretch:* Repeat the last movement. While raising spine, inhale deeply and let arms slide along floor to have hands meet overhead. Curl spine to floor while arms slide down, and exhale.

Set #2: Low Back and Waist Limbering

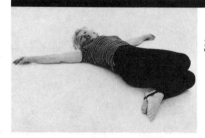

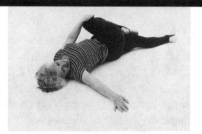

1 *Knee Drop:* Bend knees, feet on floor, legs touching. Extend arms at shoulder level with palms down. Inhale. Push both legs to floor at right, turning head to the left for balance, to stretch outside of left hip, and exhale. Change slowly several times.

2 *Open Knee Drop:* Repeat these movements with feet hip-width apart. Pushing toward floor with *inside* knee creates a stretch in the groin area.

3 *Knee Crossover:* Extend left arm out at shoulder level, palm down. With right leg straight, rest left foot on right knee. Place right hand on left knee, and pull knee toward floor at right, turning head for balance. Bounce knee down gently to stretch hip and hip joint. Then change.

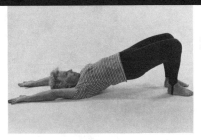

5 *Curl and Stretch:* Curl into a tight ball, arms wrapped around lower legs. Slowly uncurl, straightening legs and stretching tall. Inhale when stretching; exhale when curling up.

4 *Spine and Arm Lifting:* Repeat again, this time raising both arms through the air to touch floor overhead while spine comes up, and returning them to starting position on lowering spine.

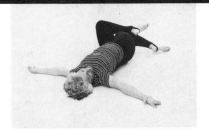

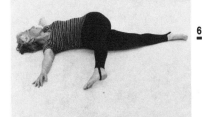

6 *Leg Circling:* From same starting position, turn right foot out and circle leg: out to the right just above floor, up, and around in a large circle to the left. Repeat several times.

4 *Pretzel Stretch:* Extend arms at shoulder level. Bend knees and cross left thigh over right, left foot touching outside of right lower leg. Slowly pull both legs toward floor at left while head turns for balance. Hold briefly before changing.

5 *Leg Crossover:* Extend arms at shoulder level with palms down. Raise straight left leg, toes pointing, and inhale. Slowly cross leg over to the right, and touch big toe to floor. Exhale. Raise leg again and inhale. Point heel up and lower leg to starting position. Exhale. Repeat twice more; then change legs.

Set #3: Low Back Stretching

1 *Knee to Chest:* Head down, draw one knee close to chest with both hands and bounce gently several times. Return leg to floor and draw other knee close.

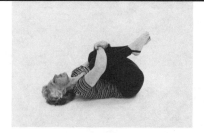

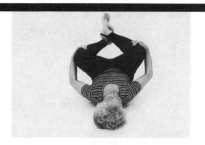

2 *Curl Up:* Draw both knees to chest, hands on shins, and rock gently.

3 *Variation:* With ankles crossed, draw knees toward outsides of chest, one hand around each knee. Lift head to stretch whole spine.

Set #4: Total Body Stretch

1 *Alternate Arm Reach:* Legs together, hold arms overhead with elbows slightly bent. Straighten right arm, reaching high to stretch waistline and rib cage, and inhale. Exhale, bending right elbow to relax. Repeat, stretching up with left arm, and alternate slowly and rhythmically with deep breathing.

2 *Arm and Leg Stretch:* From same starting position, stretch tall with right arm while pushing right heel away. Let left side relax. Change, always inhaling when stretching, exhaling when relaxing.

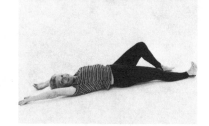

5 *Double Leg and Hip Stretch:* Bring knees to chest. Extend both legs straight up, hands behind calves, head up. Pull legs toward face, hips coming away from floor. Hold this stretch briefly; then bend knees and relax. Repeat several times.

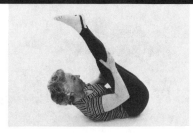

6 *Long Body Stretch:* Lie with arms overhead. Stretch very tall, pushing heels away, and inhale. Work at feeling very thin, waist and abdominal muscles long. Relax arms and legs, exhale, and repeat again.

4 ***Leg Extension:*** Draw one knee close with both hands. Extend leg straight up, hands behind knee to stretch hamstring muscles. Let go with hands, and point heel up to stretch calf muscles. Bend knee into chest again, and repeat once more with same leg before changing.

5 ***Double Leg Extension:*** Repeat above exercise, bending and stretching both legs.

3 ***Calf Stretch:*** With arms along body and toes of right foot pointed, slowly raise straight leg as high as possible, and inhale. Now point heel up, and lower the leg in flexed foot position to stretch calf. Exhale.

4 ***Hamstring Stretch:*** Raise right leg high, and place hands behind upper leg. Lift head and shoulders and gently pull straight leg toward face. Hold briefly to stretch.

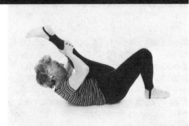

Cont.

partner exercises

Set #1: Abdominal Strength

<u>1</u>   ***Bent-Knee Sit-Ups:*** Partner A lies on back, knees bent and feet on floor, arms out at shoulder level. Partner B kneels on good padding and firmly grasps A's ankles to give strong support. A curls up, swinging arms forward and overhead to stretch tall, then returns to floor, spine round, bringing arms out again.

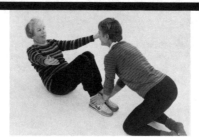 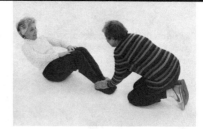

<u>2</u>   ***Progression #1:*** Partners assume same body positions, but A's hands are on thighs and stay there, eliminating the arm swinging that makes sit-ups easier. A curls down to floor, chin close to chest, hands sliding along thighs, then curls up slowly and touches fingertips to knees.

Set #2: Upper Back and Shoulder Strength

<u>1</u>   ***Trunk Raising:*** A lies face down. B kneels and firmly holds A's ankles. With chin on hands, A slowly raises head, arms, and upper body enough to feel upper back muscles and buttocks contract, holding position briefly before slowly lowering chest to floor. Repeat three times. Good padding is a must for these exercises.

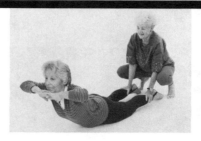 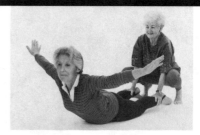

<u>2</u>   ***Progression #1:*** Arms extended at shoulder level, palms down, A again raises and lowers trunk three times very slowly and with control, making sure not to overextend the lower back.

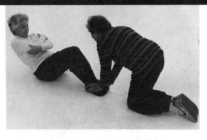

3 *Progression #2:* A's hands hold upper arms, slowly curling down and back up with this arm position. Strong ankle support is essential for this more difficult sit-up.

4 *Lifeline:* A sits with arms overhead, ankles held firmly. Holding the imaginary rope overhead, A curls spine to floor, lowering hands one by one along the rope. A then pulls up with hand-over-hand gripping.

5 Now it's the ankle holder's turn to repeat these progressive sit-up exercises.

3 *Progression #2:* Arms out, A draws slow arm circles, front to back, as trunk lifts and lowers five times. A inhales on lifting trunk, exhales on lowering.

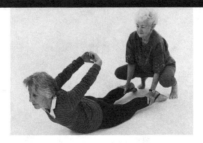

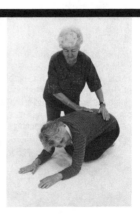

4 *Progression #3:* Hands held behind back, A raises head and trunk, pulls straight arms away from back, and inhales. A then lowers trunk and exhales.

5 *Back Massage:* A comes to a kneeling position and sits back on heels, curling up with arms relaxed along legs. B kneels at A's side and firmly massages back muscles, moving up and down along the spine from shoulder blades to hips.

Set #3: Stretching

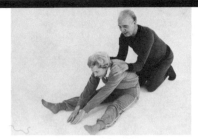

1 *Straddle Stretch:* A sits with legs comfortably apart. B kneels behind A, palms on partner's upper back, and gently pushes A's trunk forward with small pulsing movements. A reaches forward with long arms.

2 *Variation:* B stands in front and holds A's hands, pulling partner forward to stretch.

3 *Straight Leg Stretch:* A sits with legs straight and together, hands relaxed on floor. B pushes gently from behind, hands on upper back.

Set #4: Waist and Trunk Stretching

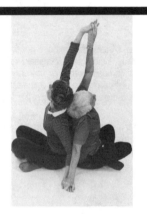 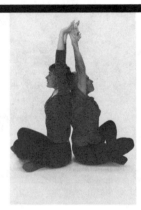

1 *Single Arm Lift:* Partners sit back to back, legs crossed, backs touching, and hold hands. They place one set of hands to floor near hips, raise other arms out and overhead slowly, and inhale while reaching tall. After lowering arms and exhaling, they then reach high with other arms.

2 *Double Arm Lift:* In same position, partners slowly raise all arms out and overhead. They inhale deeply, stretch very tall, hands meeting overhead. Their arms lower slowly as they exhale.

Set #5: Sit Up and Stretch

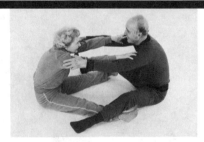 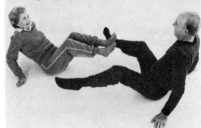

1 *Curl Up/Stretch:* Sitting facing each other, legs straight and together, partners stretch arms forward and try to touch each other's fingertips. Tucking chin close to chest, hands on legs, they slowly curl spine to floor. Both try to curl up again (with a bit of struggling), and reach out to touch each other. Repeat several times.

2 *Sit Up and Hug:* Legs apart now, partners reach forward with long arms and try to hug each other, placing hands on partner's upper arms or shoulders. Then, with arms extended forward, they slowly curl spines to floor and lie down. Repeat.

3 *Leg Circling:* Partners sit facing each other, A's legs about 1 ft apart, and B's legs between A's, feet at each other's knee level. Leaning back, hands behind hips for good support, they lift both legs and try to circle them around each other: 3 circles one way, 3 the other way.

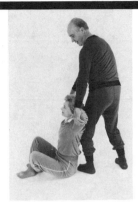

4 *Spine Straightener:* A sits with legs crossed, hands behind head. B stands sideways behind A, providing firm support by bracing the spine with outside of lower leg, holding partner's elbows. B pulls A's elbows back, straightening partner's spine and stretching chest and shoulders.

5 *Low Back Stretch:* A sits with legs crossed, hands on floor in front. B pushes gently against partner's upper back to bring upper body forward between legs while A's hands slide forward along floor.

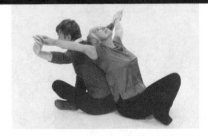

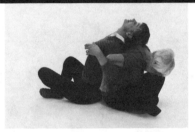

6 *Back Massage:* Partners stay in cross-legged position, backs touching, hands on floor next to hips. Both wriggle vigorously, massaging each other's backs, trying to make contact with all parts of the back while wriggling.

3 *Chest Stretch:* Partners hold hands and extend arms out at shoulder level. A pulls B's arms forward, bouncing gently several times, and then it's B's turn to help A stretch. Keeping spines erect, they brace each other for this stretch.

5 *Variation:* Partners link elbows, backs touching. They slowly rock back and forth, one person bending forward between open knees while the other arches back a little, supported by partner's back.

4 *Progression:* Repeat this exercise, but have A bend forward a little this time as B arches back and looks up, supported by partner's back. B then bends forward to let A stretch.

4 *Tandem Bike:* Both lean back on lower arms, soles of feet firmly connecting with partner's. They keep enough distance between them to be able to bicycle together, feet moving through the air.

5 *Wide Leg Stretch:* Partners keep same upper body positioning. With feet touching, they raise legs straight up. Legs slowly open wide to stretch insides of thighs. Close legs, and repeat several times.

7
endurance activities

Always lively and fun, this part of each class offers the greatest variety of activities and movement patterns. Energy is generated and calories are burned; it's the time for putting a bit of sweat back into everyone's life.

Brisk walking patterns are good activities with which to start the endurance segment of a class. They demand enough exertion to increase heart rate and breathing but are not too demanding. There are many variations of walking to improve coordination and involve the whole body in rhythmical, large-muscle movements. Instead of walking in circles, start at one end of the room and walk across, practicing a new step on the way over and perfecting it on the way back. Or you may want to divide the class into two groups, each using half of the room, and have them walk toward each other. If the class is large, you can form four groups, one for each corner of the room, and walk diagonally. Group 1 starts, and when these folks arrive in the middle, Group 2 to their right can start. When this group reaches the middle, the first group has arrived in Group 3's corner, and they can now take off. Each group needs a leader who knows when to start walking to keep confusion at a minimum.

Alternate easy steps with more demanding ones, and always think about variety to keep participants from becoming either fatigued or bored. Participants often generate new ideas for additional steps and patterns. If someone has a suggestion, have that person lead the group across.

You may want to start the endurance segment of your class with a brisk walk around the block, adding a variety of arm movements. Walk purposefully, upper body erect, chin up, breathing deeply, and smiling happily. Walk either in a large circle or in individual patterns using all available space. Suggest walking in large figure-8 patterns, zig-zagging the width of the room or changing direction often. As participants move in their own patterns, they encounter the rest of the class along the way to say hello, shake hands, or link arms with someone to march on. This is a good time for exchanging the latest news. Monitor the group, and offer your arm to someone who needs support.

Walking pace is determined by the music you select. Walk briskly to a strong, invigorating beat. Arm movements provide upper body exercise and increase heart rate and breathing.

walking patterns

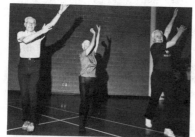

6 While looking at hands, swing both arms over right shoulder on two steps, over left on two.

7 Fists at shoulders, alternate arms for punching movement toward ceiling. Take two steps for each arm straightening and bending. Then punch with both arms on two steps; return fists to shoulders on two.

8 Reach straight ahead next, and do opposites: right arm reaches as left leg steps forward. Pull elbow back sharply. Make it snappy, one arm movement for each step.

9 Alternate arms for large arm circles from front to back on each two steps.

10 Extend arms out at shoulder level. With each four walking steps, lower arms, cross and circle up and around, wrists crossing overhead.

11 Begin with arms down. Swing arms forward and up, then down and out to shoulder level on each four steps.

12 Raise arms out to sides and overhead on two steps; lower them on the next two.

1 Extend arms at shoulder level. Cross and open straight arms for each two walking steps.

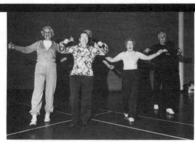

2 Push elbows back at shoulder level; then open arms wide. Take four steps for each complete arm pattern.

3 Clap hands twice in front, twice behind body, two claps for each two steps. Change to clapping once in front, once behind body, one clap for each step.

4 Combine these patterns to work on coordination:
  a) Clap twice in front, twice behind body, taking four steps.
  b) Clap once in front, once behind body, twice, taking four more steps.

5 Hold hands at chest. On two steps, fling right arm out at shoulder level and return hand to chest. Repeat with left arm on next two steps.

13 Hold hands to raise arms forward and overhead on two steps; lower them on two.

14 Arms move in breaststroke pattern on each four steps.

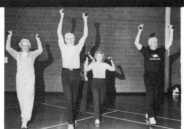

Everyone will be much warmer and breathing deeply after several minutes of some of these brisk movements. Bring the group to the end of the room now to practice some steps together.

Add your own, and your students', ideas to this list. There's no limit if you use your imagination. Once your group is in better condition, you can repeat some of these arm movements holding 1- or 2-lb dumbbells while walking.

Set #1

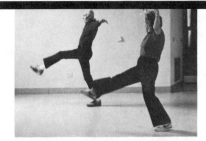

1 *Circus Horse Prance:* Roll from ball to heel of each foot, knees loose, for foot and calf exercise. Keep feet low and body erect, chin straight ahead.

2 *High Stepper:* Arms wide for balance, lift knee high with each step as if clearing an obstacle.

3 *Long Steps:* Try to get across the room with as few long steps as possible. Repeat several times to improve.

Set #2:

1 *Pigeon-Toed Walk:* Turn feet in and stomp with heavy steps.

2 *Charlie Chaplin Walk:* Turn feet out and take small running steps, keeping legs stiff.

3 *Combination:* Do four of each. Don't trip.

4 *Energetic Walk:* Smile as you take long steps, your posture erect, arms swinging very energetically.

5 *Tight Walk:* Walk on toes, and contract your buttock, abdominal, and leg muscles. Only arms are relaxed. Walk across room with stiff legs, working at abdominal lift and feeling tall.

Set #3

1 *Tall Walk:* On toes, arms overhead. Reach tall with right arm on two steps, with left arm on two.

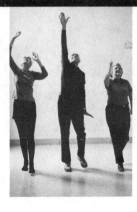

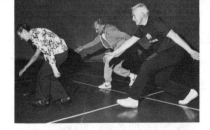

2 *Monkey Walk:* Slump forward, arms hanging, hands close to floor, knees bent. Swing arms in scissor pattern while walking in this crouch position, one arm swing for each two steps.

4 *Toe Touch Walk:* Walk lightly, testing floor with each step by touching ball of foot to floor before placing full weight on it: It's touch-step, touch-step. Arms swing over right shoulder as right leg steps forward, over left shoulder as left leg steps forward.

6 *Swivel Walk:* Arms wide, walk on balls of feet. Turn right foot in, step in front of left foot, swivel hips, and step forward with left foot. This movement comes from the hip joints and propels you forward with a strong swivel motion.

7 *Hip Wagger:* Walk, swinging hips from side to side, feet hip-width apart. Knees are relaxed, and hip joints generate this movement.

3 *Happy Walk:* On toes, back very straight, chin up, chest out. Walk with a bounce in your step.

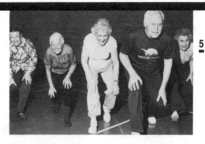

5 *Side Steps:* Right hip leading, take large steps sideways halfway across room. Turn body and continue with left leg leading. Repeat, holding hands with a partner.

4 *Knee-Bend Walk:* With feet hip-width apart, hands on thighs, try to get across room with knees bent enough to give thigh muscles a good workout.

Set #4:

1 ***Fencer's Walk:*** Walk backwards, arms out for balance. Swing right leg out, and take a big step behind left foot, shifting weight to right foot. Repeat, swinging left leg out and behind you. To avoid stepping on each other's toes, don't let everyone start at the same time.

2 ***Lame Leg Step:*** Walk, pulling right stiff leg behind you, working hard with left leg. Walk back across room dragging left leg.

3 ***Combination:*** Take four walking steps, then drag right leg for four steps. Four more walking steps and drag left leg. (This is similar to the old-fashioned kids' scooters, which were pushed along this way). Repeat with partner, coordinating feet, then in rows of six.

Set #5: Coordination Steps

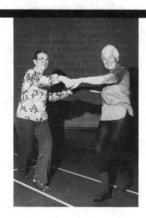

1 ***Grapevine:*** Walk across room sideways with the grapevine step, arms held out at shoulder level with elbows lightly bent. Knees are relaxed, and hips swivel to move across room easily and gracefully. Try this step slowly for a lap, then a little faster, feeling loose and relaxed. Repeat with partner.

2 ***Walk and Grapevine Combination:*** Walk forward four steps. Still facing forward, take four grapevine steps to the right, starting with the nonweightbearing foot. Again, walk forward; then grapevine to the left. Practice slowly first.

Set #6: The Handshake Circle

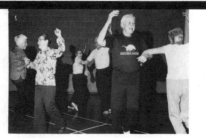 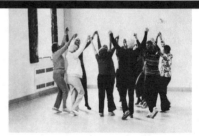

Bring the group into a large circle. Each person takes a partner. Have them hold right hands, facing each other in single circle formation. Practice without music first. When the group starts to move, partners walk away from each other, their left hands free to reach for the free left hand of the person coming toward them. Weaving past each other, once on the inside, then on the outside of the circle, the group moves along briskly, shaking right, then left hands. Depending on the music you select, participants can walk briskly, skip lightly, or move along with a polka step, always reaching for the next outstretched hand. Those with contra-dance experience know this circle formation and can help clear the confusion that initially ensues.

Go around the circle twice (keep going when meeting partner for the first time). The second time around, link arms with partner and swing around a few times to the right, then a few times to the left. Then form a large circle, hold hands, walk or skip into the circle lifting all arms high, and walk or skip back again lowering arms. Repeat several times.

4 **Heel Walk:** Walk across room on heels to stretch calf muscles.

5 **Toe Walk:** Walk on toes, tall and proudly.

6 **Combination:** Walk on toes for four steps, on heels for four.

7 **Long and Short Steps:** Take four long, slow steps, then eight quick, short running steps.

3 **Stretch and Bend:** Take four walking steps on toes with arms overhead, four steps in Monkey Walk.

Set #7: Snake Dance

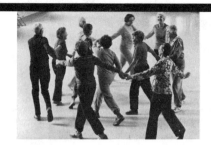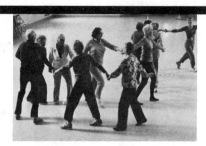

First, clearly explain what you plan to do to eliminate a lot of unnecessary confusion and possible frustration. All participants hold hands in a large circle. The leader lets go of one hand and briskly walks along the inside of the circle, pulling everyone else along in single file. Keep going in circles that become smaller and smaller, forming a coil, until there is no space left in the center. Everyone continues holding hands while turning to face out and uncoil, walking in enlarging circles until the pattern is dissolved.

Set #8: Leg Swinging in Connected Circle for Improved Balance

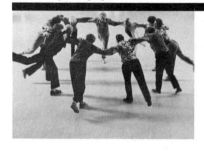

In circle formation, have participants place their hands on each other's nearest shoulder (not around neck) for balance and support. Choose music appropriate for swinging movements; a moderate waltz beat is nice. Emphasize complete movements instead of speed. Have everyone raise the left knee. Keeping the leg relaxed and loose, they swing it across body from right to left and back. Give clear instructions while demonstrating to make sure that all legs swing to the same side at the same time. After 10 complete swings, let go of each other's shoulders and make a quarter turn to the right.

With arms out for balance, continue this leg swinging from right to left and back, without support now, still standing on the right leg. This feels and looks a bit more unsteady than the balanced circle and will cause everyone to hop around for balance. Connect the circle again and repeat all this, swinging the right leg.

Set #9: The Grand March

Participants enjoy doing this pattern to brisk, peppy music. Start at one end of the room and walk across energetically in *single file*, one behind the other. You might want to stand at the other end to direct traffic. As they approach, the first person goes to the right, the next to the left, the third to the right, and so on until two single files are walking back along the long walls of the room. They meet in pairs and walk down the middle toward you again where the first couple turns right, the second left, and so on. At the head of the room, two couples will join and walk across in fours. They finish in rows of eight, linking arms, and reverse pattern.

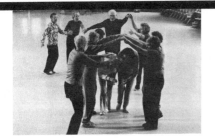 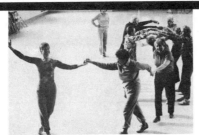

At this point, form a tunnel: The first two in line (leader and next person) hold hands and raise their arms. The next two go through, hold hands, and stand beside the first pair. Continue this pattern till everyone has ducked through the arch and added to it. The arch can now be unravelled by having the couple who started the formation walk through, holding hands, and taking the other couples along as their turn comes. The last person in line always reaches for a hand belonging to the last couple in the arch until everyone is connected again in single file. Everyone continues walking, forming a circle again to finish.

Next, hold hands in the circle and start swinging the left leg forward and back. Start low, slowly increasing height of the lift and involving the whole body more. Those who feel secure enough can try these forward and back swings next without holding on, keeping arms out at shoulder level for balance. Repeat, swinging the right leg, all legs moving together.

These are large movements involving large muscle groups, and everyone will be very warm and a bit breathless. Make sure to monitor your group throughout these activities, adjusting your demonstration according to signals you receive.

Hold hands now, standing close to each other in the circle. Lift all arms high, bend back a little to look up, and take a deep breath. Next, bend knees and bring all hands to floor while exhaling forcefully. Repeat 10 times, 5 fast, 5 slow.

Set #10: Alley Cat

The Alley Cat is still popular with all ages at Polish weddings and is best done, of course, to Alley Cat music. Divide the class into straight rows facing you, and turn your back to the class to demonstrate the following steps:

1 Right foot steps out lightly, back to center, twice. Repeat with left foot.

2 Right foot steps back, returns to center, twice. Repeat with left foot.

3 Right knee lifts across toward left shoulder, foot touches down lightly, twice. Place weight on right foot now and repeat knee lifts with left leg.

Set #11: Walking With Dowel

1 *Prance:* Place dowel behind shoulder blades for good posture and prance across.

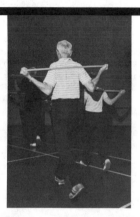

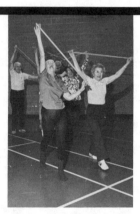

2 *Tall Walk:* On toes, dowel behind shoulder blades. Walk very tall and with a spring in each step.

3 *Arm Lifting:* Walk briskly, raising dowel overhead on two steps, lowering it on the next two.

Set #12: Partner Walks With Dowel

1 *Arm Lifting:* Partners walk side by side, holding dowel low in front. They raise arms high on two steps, lower them on the next two.

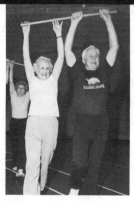

2 *Draw a Square:* As in Set #11, partners work together for a perfect square.

3 *Push and Pull:* As in Set #11, partners step forward with the same leg at the same time, lifting and lowering arms, taking four steps for each complete arm pattern.

4 Right leg kicks across to the left once, foot returns to floor, and left leg kicks across once.

5 Hop in place once, clapping hands.

6 Hop again, clapping, while making a quarter turn to the right with this hop.

7 Stay in this new position to repeat the whole pattern, hopping a quarter turn to the right again each time the sequence ends. Repeat until music ends.

4 *Progression:* For each four walking steps, raise dowel overhead, touch it behind shoulder blades, raise arms again, and lower them to touch thighs in front.

5 *Draw a Square:* For each four walking steps, draw a large square with dowel: Arms low, push dowel to the right, lift it high at right, overhead to left, and lower it at left.

6 *Push and Pull:* Push dowel forward at chest level on two steps; pull it toward chest on the next two.

7 *Progression:* To this push and pull, add raising and lowering arms, taking four walking steps for these two arm patterns.

4 *March and Kick:* Starting with the right foot, partners take three walking steps (right, left, right), then kick the left leg toward dowel on the fourth step. Continue, kicking right leg next.

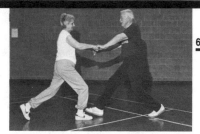

6 *Grapevine:* Facing each other and holding dowel at chest level, partners travel sideways with the grapevine step. Have them work at coordinating steps and swiveling hips. They return with other leg leading.

5 *Backward Walk:* Partners face each other and hold dowel at chest level. They walk across, one person walking forward, the other backward. Caution them to not step on each other's toes by staying a safe distance away from each other and coordinating legs. They return in same position so the other person walks backward now.

Set #13: Waltzing

Teach the waltz step at a moderate pace. Emphasize the long first step, bending knees deeply, then the two steps in place on toes: One-two-three is the count, step one being the long emphasis step forward, two and three being light steps in place. Most seniors know how to dance the waltz and love these practices. Swing scarves for graceful movement. Demonstrate the following steps:

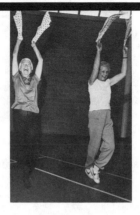

1 Waltz across singly, arms swinging in opposition to legs, for balance and graceful movement.

2 Standing side by side, waltz with a partner. Hold inside hands and swing arms forward and up on three steps, down and back a little on three.

Set #14: Light Hopping and Kicking in Place

1 *Run in Place:* Lift feet only a few inches away from floor. Elbows are bent at sides, and arms move comfortably.

2 *Hop in Place:* Lightly hop twice on right foot, twice on left foot.

3 *Hop-Kick:* Turn the second hop into a relaxed forward swing of the nonweightbearing lower leg, kicking an imaginary ball. Alternate feet, scissor swinging arms in opposition.

Set #15: Prancing and Hopping in Rows

Form rows of eight, and place hands on each other's nearest shoulders. Try to keep rows straight while moving across.

1 *Prance:* Prance in good posture, lifting knees. Everyone starts with the same foot. foot.

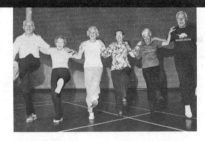

2 *Hop Across:* While moving forward, everyone hops lightly on right foot twice, then on left foot twice.

3 Waltz alone again, increasing the arm swing: very high on three steps, way back on three while bending forward with round upper back.

4 Increase tempo and lift for a light, vigorous waltzing across.

5 Hold hands in rows of eight and waltz across, swinging arms forward and back.

6 Finish by forming a circle, holding hands, and waltzing into and out of the circle with arm swinging.

4 *Run-Kick:* Take three light running steps in place, and kick lower leg forward on four: run-two-three/kick right leg, run-two-three/kick left leg.

5 *Circle Hop:* Hop-kick a circle to the right, a circle to the left, and finish with easy jogging in place.

3 *Hop-Kick Forward:* On second hop, everyone kicks one lower leg forward with relaxed knee. The pattern is hop-kick right, hop-kick left. Work at kicking the same leg at the same time.

4 *Prance and Kick:* All take three prancing steps forward, knees lifting a little higher now, and one lower leg swings forward on the fourth count. Alternate leg kicking: prance-two-three/kick right, prance-two-three/kick left.

5 *Progression:* Take four prancing steps forward. Staying in place, hop lightly on right foot twice, kicking left leg forward on second hop, then hop on left foot twice, kicking right leg forward on second hop. The pattern is prance-two-three-four/hop-kick right, hop-kick left.

6 *Stiff-Legged Kicks:* All lean back slightly and move across floor, kicking legs forward stiffly, knees locked, feet close to floor.

skipping

Almost everyone remembers how to skip. Skipping is something that makes everyone feel young, light, and cheerful, and is fun to do for those reasons. A skipping step is a light double hop from one foot to the other, traveling forward, knees lifting a little with each step.

Set #16: Skipping Progression

1 *Easy Skipping:* Practice relaxed skipping to good music, arms relaxed.

2 *Knee Lift Skipping:* Skip more vigorously, lifting knees a little higher.

3 *Arm Swing Skipping:* Skip across, arms swinging in opposition: right knee up and left arm forward, left knee up and right arm forward.

7 *Partner Skipping:* Face each other and hold hands. Skip across, one forward and the other backward, taking small, light steps and coordinating feet, being careful not to step on each other's toes. Return in same position to let the other person go backward now.

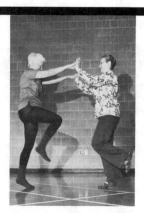

4 **_Double Arm Swing:_** Skip, swinging both arms forward, then back, one arm movement for each skipping step.

5 **_Swivel Skip:_** Turn the Swivel Walk into swivel skipping steps, arms held out at shoulder level with elbows bent.

6 **_Walk and Skip:_** With hands on hips, walk four steps, and skip four.

Cont.

polka steps

The polka step is similar to the waltz step, and most seniors know how to polka. It's a one-two-three step without the deep dip of the waltz. The first step is an energetic, long travel step bringing you forward, steps two and three are small. Knees stay relaxed throughout.

Set #17: Polka Patterns

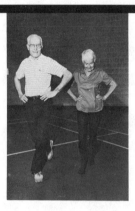

1   *Easy Polka Step:* With hands on hips, polka across room.

2   *Arm Swing Polka:* Arms swing relaxed to the right as right leg steps forward, to the left as left leg steps forward.

3   *Progression:* Polka more vigorously, swinging arms higher and taking longer steps.

Set #18: Polka Partner Patterns

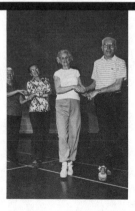

1   *Hand Holding:* Hold inside hands, swing arms forward and back, one swing for each polka step forward, and coordinate leg movement.

2   *Crossing Hand Hold:* Side by side, hold hands in front, arms crossed. Polka in zig-zag pattern at an open angle to the right, then to the left, same legs leading.

3   *Progression:* Move more energetically, trying to get across with as few polka steps as possible.

4   *Polka Turn:* Without hand-holding, partners move forward side by side, hands behind back. Walk forward four steps; then turn toward each other for one polka step, away from each other for a second polka step. Walk forward again.

4   Scissor Arms: Swing arms in opposition to polka steps.

5   Zig-Zag Polka: Hands behind back, polka diagonally to the right, right leg leading, with one step, then out to the left, left leg leading, to move across in a zig-zag pattern.

6   Polka Turn: Hands behind back, right shoulder facing forward, take one polka step and make a one-half turn so that left shoulder now faces direction of movement. Continue moving forward, right and left shoulder leading alternately.

7   Open Arm Polka Turn: Arms extended at shoulder level, polka across with these half turns, right, then left arm leading.

8   Walk and Polka: Take four walking steps, then two polka steps forward, combining for a count of eight. This pattern is fun to practice without music. Everyone becomes very quiet, listening to footsteps and concentrating on working together for perfection.

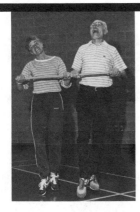

Single and partner skipping and polka patterns are fun with dowels, too. Even though steps are the same, they seem different when practicing with hand equipment. Add them for occasional variety: skipping and polkaing with dowel behind shoulder blades, swinging dowel from side to side, sharing dowel with a partner, and so on. Be creative. Find new ways of moving, but try everything out at home before taking your ideas into the classroom.

light running

When we run, emphasis is always on staying light on our feet, taking small steps, and keeping feet low to eliminate jarring and to avoid overexertion. We are not preparing for foot races, and everyone knows when to slow to a brisk walk if running becomes too tiring. If you are a committed runner yourself, make sure to hold back as you lead your class: Take small, light steps because everyone will watch and follow your example. On the whole, there is greater variety with walking, skipping, waltzing, and polka steps, but light running adds another option. If using music, make sure the beat is neither too fast nor too slow; either way, running will become too tiring. Choose music that will encourage light, comfortable running.

Set #19: Serpentine Run

Start in single file at one end of the room, lightly running back and forth across width of room. Lead the way, setting the right pace with your demonstration. Keep loops narrow so that it takes a while to reach the other end of the room. In this pattern, participants see each other coming and going, which creates a colorful movement pattern. When you reach the other end, continue running along wall, opening up the serpentine and bringing everyone into a large circle. Finish with easy jogging in place.

Set #21: Endurance Work With Chair Support

Chair support helps those with weak legs and ankles to feel more secure with light hopping and jumping activities. Less stress is placed on joints when some of the body's weight is absorbed by holding on to the chair back.

1 **Run in Place:** Stand behind chair, hands on chair back. Lightly run in place.

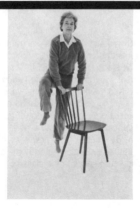

2 **Hopping:** Lightly hop twice on right foot, twice on left foot.

3 **Side-to-Side Hop:** With feet together, hop lightly to the right. Take a second light hop in place; then hop to the left.

4 **Side Leg Kicks:** Lightly hop in place on both feet once, and swing left leg out on second hop. Hop in place again on both feet, and swing right leg out next.

5 **Legs Apart and Together:** Lightly jump to bring legs apart, hop in place once, jump to bring legs together, and hop in place again.

Set #20: Sprinter's Run

Divide class into groups of five, standing in single file one behind the other. Spread out the groups and begin light running around the room. While running at a comfortable pace with small steps, the fifth runner passes his or her group on the inside, sprinting for a few seconds, and becomes the group's leader. As soon as the fifth runner takes the lead position, the last person in the group passes to the front of the line. Continue this running and passing pattern for the length of your music selection, the passing person always having to readjust steps again when taking the lead position. Keep enough distance between groups, and make sure each group stays together.

Passing on the outside requires a longer sprint and becomes too demanding. Those unable to run can form their own group and participate at a walking pace, walking very briskly to pass.

<u>6</u> *Scissor Jump:* Staying light on feet, hop to bring one leg back, the other forward, and continue this scissor pattern, always adding a second little hop in place.

<u>8</u> Finish with easy jogging in place.

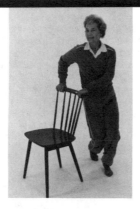

<u>7</u> *Hip Swivel Twist:* Legs together, rise onto balls of feet. Bend knees a little and swivel hips, pushing knees from side to side while lowering body into a half knee bend. Continue to swivel as you come up again.

Set #22: Dowel Serpentine

Place dowels in two long rows on floor, leaving about 6 ft between each dowel. Divide class into two single file lines and run lightly in small serpentine pattern around dowels, weaving in and out, leaning into curves and lifting outside arms high in each curve. Return, running along second row of dowels.

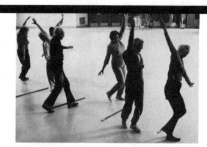

3 Take small running steps between dowels; then hop over each with both feet. Lift feet high enough to clear dowel.

4 For coordination practice, place dowels unequal distances apart so that steps have to be adjusted for light running.

5 Cool down by walking across, lifting knee high to step over each dowel as if it were a giant obstacle.

Set #24: Dowel Catch in Circle

Each person has a dowel. Form a circle, right shoulders facing out, standing one behind the other, about 3 ft apart. Place one end of dowel to floor at right, right hand lightly holding other end. Explain the activity first: Run forward quickly, letting go of your own dowel and catching the one in front before it falls. The leader gives the starting command, calling "Ready, set, GO!" as everyone lets go of their dowel and quickly moves forward to catch the next one. Problems present themselves instantly: Some hang on to their own dowel while running for the other, others throw their dowel behind themselves, and so on. On the whole, there is a lot of noise as most of the dowels fall to the floor with great crashing sounds. Don't spend too much time with this; stop before it becomes less than fun.

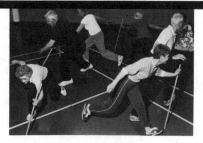

Set #23: Dowel Obstacle Course

Place dowels on floor as you did for the Dowel Serpentine. Divide into two groups, starting at opposite ends of room.

1 Run lightly in single file with small steps, clearing each dowel.

2 Run lightly between dowels, and take a little jump over each, pushing off with one foot. Don't rush each other, and make every effort to clear each dowel. If a dowel starts to roll, everyone should stop for a few seconds until it's put back in place. Work at light, feathery jumps.

Cont.

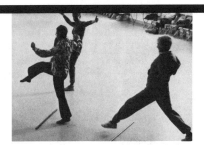

cooling down
with dowels and partners

Spend a few minutes with partner exercises
to cool down and stretch.

Set #25: Partners Sharing One Dowel

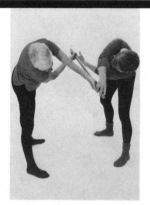
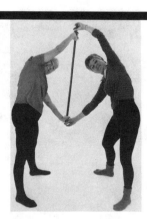

1 *Long Back Stretch:* Stand across from
each other, holding dowel. Step away until
back and arms are long and stretched, pulling aginst dowel. Push hips far back and
gently bounce chest toward floor.

2 *Side Bending:* Stand facing each other,
with legs well apart, dowel held horizontally.
Slowly bend to one side, raising one set of
arms high overhead while other hands push
dowel across lower body.

3 *High Side Bending:* Same position, with all
arms high, bend comfortably from side to
side. Add a little bounce to each stretch before changing.

Set #26: Sitting Stretches, Sharing One Dowel

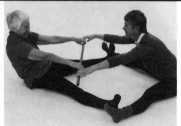

1 *Rocking Stretch:* Sit facing each other,
legs comfortably apart, and hold dowel.
Rock back and forth slowly: Partner A leans
back, pulling B forward for a good stretch of
back and leg muscles. Hold each position
for a few seconds before changing.

2 *Coffee Grinder:* Use same leg position.
Progress to circling of upper bodies, going
as far in each direction as possible. Circle
several times each way, moving slowly to
avoid dizziness.

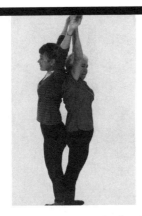

4 ***Chest Stretch:*** Stand back to back, spines touching. Hold dowel overhead, hands shoulder-width apart. One partner pulls the other's arms forward to stretch chest and shoulders with gentle bouncing. Change.

3 ***Dowel Rolling:*** Partner A puts dowel on floor between legs and rolls it forward toward B, keeping fingertips on dowel as long as possible before B takes it and rolls it back.

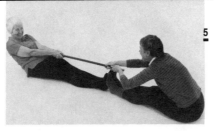

5 ***Dowel Sit-Up:*** Turn this stretch into a combination of stretches and sit-ups. A allows B to curl spine to floor very slowly, keeping back round and chin close to chest. A has to come forward to lower B to floor. B now curls up from floor with as little help as possible from partner and bends forward to lower A to floor.

4 ***Straight Leg Stretch:*** Sit with legs together and straight, soles of feet touching. Hold dowel the long way to make this stretch possible. A rocking motion starts again with A leaning back and pulling B forward gently. This is not a power contest; allow each person to stretch comfortably. Since feet are braced, calves and heelcords are included in this stretch.

Set #27: Partners Sharing Two Dowels

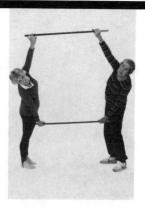

1 **_Dowel Lifting:_** Stand facing each other, legs together, arms at sides. Share two dowels, holding one end in each hand. Raise both dowels out to sides and high overhead, rising onto toes and inhaling. Lower arms and heels, exhaling.

2 **_Single Arm Sidebending:_** Stand with legs well apart, facing each other. Bend upper body to one side, lifting the opposite arms high and close to ears. Other arms hang low and relaxed. Alternate bending from side to side, adding a little bounce to each stretch.

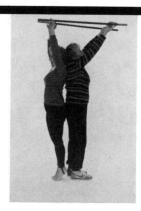

4 **_Back to Back Dowel Lifting:_** Stand back to back, legs together, arms down. Raise one dowel out and overhead, bringing arms close to ears. As arms lower, raise the other dowel high.

5 **_Double Arm Lifting:_** In same position, raise both dowels so they touch overhead. Inhale. Lower arms to sides and exhale.

3 **Dowel Swinging:** Stand a safe distance apart, legs apart. Swing dowels from side to side, pushing off with feet and light knee bending. Swing dowels a little higher each time, and end up adding a little jump to each swing.

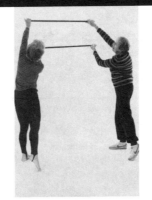 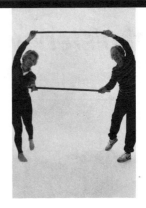

Cont.

6 **Chin-Up With Dowels:** Three people of equal height and weight work together, and each threesome needs two dowels. Two persons stand facing each other, holding both dowels at each end with a firm grip. Third person sits on the floor, hips directly under dowels, legs straight and together, back straight, and hands gripping dowels firmly. The carriers stand with legs apart and knees slightly bent to carry the sitter's weight. The sitter attempts to raise hips away from floor by bending elbows and bringing chin toward dowels. For most, raising the hips just a few inches is difficult enough, and for some the attempt may become the exercise. Try several times before the other two take turns.

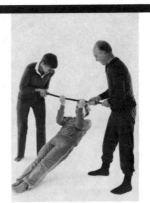

upholstery webbing bands

Set #28: Carousel

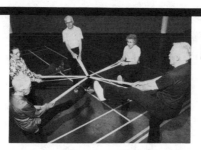

The class separates into groups of five. Each person takes one band, and each group needs one metal ring. Form a circle, facing in, and pull all bands through this ring. Place one hand through each loop. The group is now connected. Step back to make bands taut.

1 *High Leg Kicks:* All five kick the right, then the left leg up, starting low, then higher, to bring foot to band.

2 *Crossover Step and Kick:* All step right with right foot, left foot steps across right in front; right foot steps right again, and left leg kicks across to the right. Return left foot to floor, cross right foot over left, step left with left foot, and kick right leg across. The pattern is step, cross, step, kick. Everyone has to work together, doing the same thing at the same time, which takes a little practice. Being connected as a group helps those with coordination problems.

3 *Grapevine:* Lean back a little, arms stretched long and relaxed. Practice the grapevine step going around to the right a few times, then to the left, all feet doing the same thing at the same time. Practice with more knee bending and hip swiveling for smooth, graceful moving in circles.

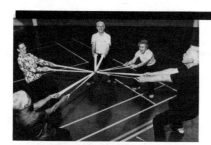

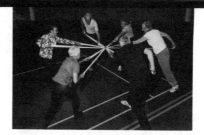

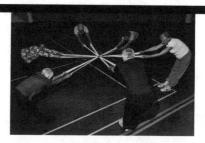

5 *Water-Skiers:* Stand facing in, legs apart. Bend knees, tucking hips under, upper body leaning back. Knees push forward to feel weight on thighs. Stretch arms long. Bounce in this waterskiing position 10 times; then straighten legs to relax for a few seconds, and repeat once more.

6 *See-Saw:* Stand facing in, legs apart, upper body forward, with one hand through each loop. Pull one elbow back to stretch other arm forward, and alternate, moving arms briskly in this see-saw pattern. Coordinate arm movements, move hips from side to side, and keep knees loose.

7 *Back and Leg Stretch:* Finish by stepping away until back is flat, arms stretched long. Push hips back for a good stretch.

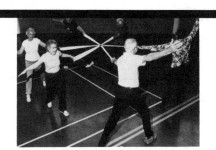

4 *Skipping:* All turn sideways, left shoulder facing in, left hand through both loops. Arm is stretched, body weight out, so there is tension on all bands. The group skips in circles a few times, then changes direction by holding bands with right hand. Repeat this pattern with polka steps and more enthusiastic swinging of outside arms. This can turn into a speedy merry-go-round, so keep pace reasonable. Slow down by walking with long steps, outside arm swinging overhead toward center on two steps, out and down on two steps.

Cont.

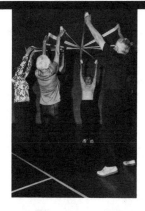

8 *Stretch and Bend:* Stand closer together now and raise all arms very high so that bands form a tight roof overhead. Inhale. Relax as you bend forward to exhale. Repeat several times.

Set #29: Floor Sitting, Groups of Five

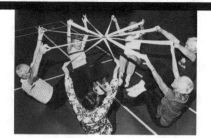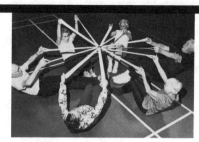

1 *Graceful Sit-Up:* Put one hand through each loop. Knees are bent, feet on floor with all toes touching in the middle. Raise arms overhead in a wide V and stretch bands to create a roof. Tuck chin to chest and round the spine, slowly curling down to floor simultaneously. While the leader counts, the groups curl up again, coming to a sitting position with spine very erect, raising arms to stretch bands overhead. Each group has to work together for smooth movements. This looks very graceful, helps everyone feel successful in doing sit-ups, and can be followed by a sit-up competition between groups, trying for 15 or 20 sit-ups depending on ability and class mood.

bicycle inner tubes

Set #30: Obstacle Run

Place all tubes on floor, evenly divided throughout room. Everyone runs lightly in individual patterns around tubes, dodging each other to avoid collisions and to work on quick reactions. Use light running music for this activity, and keep everyone moving for several minutes. Ask participants to hold hands with another person somewhere along the way and continue running as partners.

2 *Sitting See-Saw Stretch:* All legs comfortbly apart, feet touching, perform the see-saw stretching movement. Pull one elbow back while other arm stretches long and upper body moves forward between legs. Stay in each stretch for a few seconds. Then speed arm movements up a little for vigorous exercise and fun. Again, each group has to coordinate arm movements, having all right arms stretch forward at the same time. REPEAT with legs together and straight, bending forward and stretching each arm long.

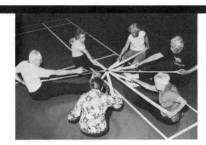

3 *Leg Lifting:* With legs slightly separated and bands held between legs, everyone in the group leans back enough to feel abdominals contract. All right legs lift and lower three times, left legs next, and now everyone tries to raise both legs at the same time. Balancing on buttocks is made easier by being anchored. Stay for a few seconds and collapse.

The last exercise is rolling each band up before it's returned to storage.

Set #31: Run and Jump

Continue light running and jump into and out of each tube along the way. Jump with right foot leading, change to left foot leading, or take light jumps into and out of tubes with feet together. Those who are tired can walk and jump. Demonstrate feathery, comfortable jumping, emphasizing feeling light on your feet. Then slow down to a walk, stepping over each tube with a giant step, knee lifting high.

Set #32: Tube Competition

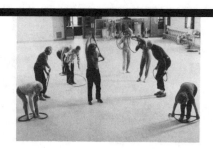

While everyone runs lightly, stop the music. This is the signal to quickly run for a tube, step into it, pick the tube up, and bring it overhead as if pulling off a sweater. Place it on the floor again, step in, repeat this action a total of three times, being as quick and agile as possible, and sit down in the tube after completing the task. Start the music again and repeat twice more. The rushing around, confusion, and laughter are great fun to watch and everyone is ready to stay down at the end for a short rest.

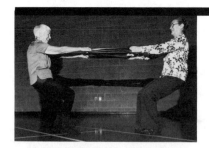
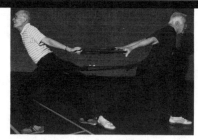
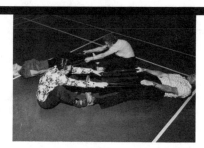

To cool down after these activities, find a partner and use two double-folded tubes. Spend a few minutes with the Water-Skiers exercise, the Long Back Stretch standing, Back-to-Back Stretch, the See-Saw Stretches sitting with legs together and straight, and some sit-ups with the help of these tubes. The stretching movements with folded tubes add elasticity for greater range of movement.

Set #33: Horse and Buggy

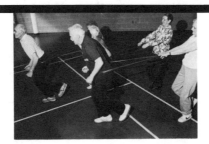

All go to one end of the room, find a partner, and use both tubes. Partner B stands behind A, who brings the tubes around pelvic area. (Tubes around the waist cause pressure against the stomach.) B holds tubes with both hands and hangs back a little, arms stretched forward. They start to run across the room with small steps, A leaning forward, elbows bent, and arms moving to help with the run. If B hangs back too much, moving forward becomes impossible. B should provide enough resistance for the "horse" in front, but exertion should be kept at a reasonable level. Change positions at the other end and go back and forth to peppy music several times. This exercise simulates an uphill run and results in huffing, puffing, and tired legs. Everyone can adjust the level of de-

mand by communicating with partner. And again, those who need to work less hard can walk briskly instead of running or sit to watch if this activity is too demanding.

Cont.

beanbags

Set #34: Beanbag Tossing

Stand in two rows about 10 feet apart, facing each other. Each person needs a partner to work with, and, to start, only one beanbag is tossed between two people. Keep all other beanbags in their storage container, not on the floor as obstacles.

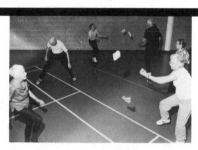

1 *Easy Toss:* Toss beanbag back and forth, tossing with right, catching with both hands. Toss in a nice arc. After some practice, test for quicker reactions by tossing straight ahead rather than high. Change to tossing with left hand, still catching with both hands.

2 *Single-Handed Toss and Catch:* Toss and catch with right hand only. (Place left hand behind back to avoid cheating on the catch.) Repeat with left hand. Don't expect to be able to stand in one spot when catching; your partner's toss may not go where you expect it. Always be prepared to move for the catch, and avoid collisions.

Set #35: Cooling Down With Partners

1 *Waist Twist:* Stand back to back, about 1 ft apart, with legs hip-width apart. Partner A holds one beanbag in both hands at waist level. Twisting strongly at the waist, beanbag is handed to B, who twists to face same direction for the exchange. Both now twist the other way, and A takes beanbag from B. Start slowly; then increase speed a little.

2 *Beanbag Push:* Sit across from partner, legs apart, beanbag on floor between legs. Partner A places both hands on beanbag and pushes it forward along floor as far as possible before B takes it and pushes it toward A.

3 *Straight Leg Forward Bending:* Sit with legs together and straight, feet touching. Partner A holds beanbag overhead, bends forward, stretches arms long, and hands the beanbag over. B now reaches tall first, then bends to hand beanbag to A again. Increase speed for fun and agility. (You may want to bring the group together for this into two straight lines facing each other, having everyone work together. Try the over-the-shoulder toss in this sitting position.)

3 *High-Arc Toss:* Toss with one hand and catch with two, tossing very high and reaching tall for the catch.

4 *Over-the-Shoulder Toss:* Take beanbag into the more coordinated hand behind lower back. Bend knees a little, round the upper back by bending forward, and try to toss the beanbag over the opposite shoulder to your partner. Keep practicing—this is not easy.

5 *Under-the-Knee Toss:* This is a little easier to accomplish. Hold beanbag in right hand, raise right knee, and toss beanbag from the outside under the knee across to partner. Coordination problems set in when this is tried with the other hand and knee.

6 *Double Beanbag Toss:* Each person holds one beanbag in right hand. Both toss simultaneously by communicating with each other and catch with the left hand. Toss with left and catch with right, establishing an even rhythm without hurrying. When you or your partner miss, start over again.

You can experiment with all these activities by initially standing closer together, then moving farther apart to make things a little more difficult. There is a great deal of bonus exercise involved in constantly retrieving stray beanbags from all over. Don't worry about beanbags hitting anyone. They frequently will, but they are light and soft. And participants usually manage instinctively to dodge those not intended for them.

4 *Sitting Waist Twist:* Sit back to back, legs crossed. Try the above waist twist in this sitting position, handing beanbag over at shoulder level.

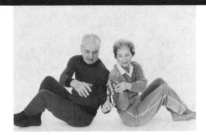

8
chair exercises

Finding a hall with a supply of sturdy, safe, armless chairs will be a real bonus to your program. Beyond being a useful piece of exercise equipment, a chair gives support, helps with balance, and is always there to sit down on to relax. Chairs should have rubber stoppers so they will not move.

In our class, bringing chairs out does not necessarily mean relaxing. Many of the exercises are quite demanding and give specific muscle groups a good workout. Even though participants benefit from staying on their feet and moving as much as possible, chairs add interesting exercise variety and are good for relaxation at the end of the class.

Chair support is very helpful to those with knee or hip problems and leg weakness. Chairs are sturdy support for getting down to and back up from the floor if physical confidence is low. Demonstrate the following steps for them:

- Stand behind chair, hands on chair back.
- Bend knees to a 90° angle.
- Lower one knee to floor, then the other.
- Place both hands on floor; you are on all fours now.
- Bring both legs to one side, sit on that hip, and straighten legs forward.

Instead of helping those who have problems, focus on the development of this body confidence and self-reliance. Many of those who live alone say that a fall with no help nearby is one of their worst fears. It is well worth spending time in your classes with these practices, both with and without chair support, to help alleviate fear and develop confidence for getting up or down safely.

exercises for the upper body

Set #1: Body Wake-Up

1 Sit comfortably, hands relaxed with open palms. Using both hands, gently slap one thigh, working your way along inside and outside of thigh to knee and back up. Lift leg and slap front and back of thigh. Finish with firm massage strokes up and down several times. Raise knee again and slap calf muscles and sides of lower leg next, moving up and back down. Finish with firm massaging.

2 Contract abdominal muscles and sit erectly. Gently slap abdominal area, outside of hips, and rib cage, ending with firm massage strokes.

3 Next, work on backs of upper arms, slapping right arm with left hand. Then grasp tissue of upper arm, and spend a little time kneading gently, moving from shoulder to elbow and back, to further increase circulation. Massage with firm strokes.

Set #2: Swimmer's Workout

1 *Crawl Stroke:* Sit with legs apart. Bend forward at waist and swim a crawl stroke, making each arm long and stretching back muscles.

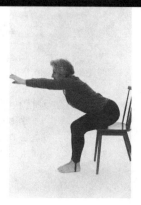 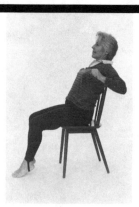

2 *Rowing:* Sit tall, arms extended forward at shoulder level. Bend forward, reach long. Pull elbows back while sitting upright again as if rowing a boat.

4 Get up and slap hips and buttocks firmly, moving hands up and down in back and along sides of hips. Slap firmly enough to cause some tingling. Slapping feels good only in padded areas: Don't slap over bony parts like shins, neck, or feet.

5 Sit with head hanging relaxed. Using all fingertips, tap skull lightly, moving from base of skull to forehead and back down several times.

6 End this body wake-up with firm massage strokes from top of legs down to feet and back, then one arm at a time from wrist to shoulder and back. This slapping, tapping, and massaging creates a warm, tingling sensation all over and makes you feel ready to spring into action.

3 *Breast Stroke:* Next, swim the breast stroke. Reach forward with both arms, fingers pointing straight ahead, upper body following arms. Now open arms wide to stretch chest while sitting upright again.

4 *Back Stroke:* Sitting tall, circle one arm at a time from front to back. Stay clear of chair by bringing arm out a little.

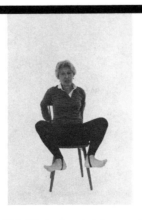 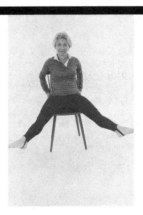

5 *Frog Kick:* Sit at edge of chair, upper back resting against chair back, arms wrapped around chair back. Raise feet a bit. Bend knees out. Then extend legs out just above floor, and bring straight legs back together, simulating the frog kick.

Set #3: Shoulders and Upper Back

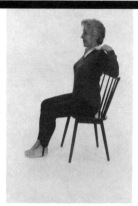

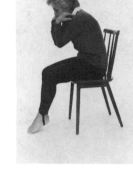

2 **Elbow to Opposite Knee:** With legs apart and hands on shoulders, bend forward and twist, touching right elbow to left knee. Sit up straight again, pushing elbows back; then touch left elbow to right knee.

1 **Elbow Touch:** Sit up straight, hands on shoulders. Push elbows back to stretch chest; then bring elbows together in front of chest, rounding and stretching shoulder girdle.

Set #4: Arm and Upper Back Strength

1 **Double Arm Push-Away:** Sit tall, chin up, arms down with palms facing back. Push straight arms back with pulsing motions, keeping them close to body. Push back 8 times, relax, and repeat.

2 **Hands Push and Pull:** Sit tall. With elbows just below shoulder level, press open palms together hard for a few seconds. Relax. Then clasp fingers and pull out hard for a few seconds. Repeat several times to strengthen arm and pectoral muscles. This is an isometric exercise, and breathing correctly is important. Inhale when relaxed; exhale while pushing or pulling.

3 **Chair Push-Away:** Sit halfway back in chair, hands grasping sides of chair seat. Place balls of feet lightly on floor. Contract abdominals and lean forward slightly. Push against chair, arms straight, and raise buttocks a few inches. Try to keep weight off feet, touching floor for balance only. Sit down and repeat several times.

Set #5: Arm and Back Strength

1 **Rocking Chair:** Sit at edge of chair, hands grasping front corners. Stand up and bring upper body forward, keeping hands on chair. Then sit down again, lean back to touch upper back to chair back, and bring both knees to chest. Turn this standing up and sitting down into a simulated rocking chair motion.

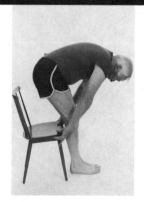

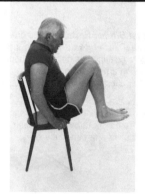

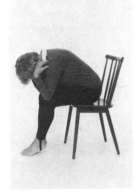

4 *Elbow Circling:* With hands on shoulders, describe front-to-back circles with elbows, starting small and enlarging circle size. Change direction.

5 *Wing Lifter:* Hands on shoulders; raise elbows out and up, feeling rib cage lift and waistline stretch. Lower elbows.

6 *Double Arm Raising:* Begin with arms relaxed at sides. Raise arms out and up, hands meeting overhead, and inhale deeply while stretching tall. Lower arms slowly and exhale.

7 *Arm Raising:* Sit up tall, spine supported by chair back, hands on thighs. Raise right arm straight and high. Push back several times, then lower arm. Repeat with left arm. Then raise both arms and push back strongly, back arching a little, and look up.

3 *Elbows to Thighs:* Legs together, hands on shoulders, push elbows back, then bend forward to touch outsides of thighs.

4 *Phantom Chair:* Sit at edge of chair, hands grasping front corners of chair seat. Raise hips and move feet forward enough for body to clear chair. Feet are directly below knees, hip-width apart. Now bend and straighten elbows to lower and raise hips in front of chair. Sit down and shake hands and arms out to relax.

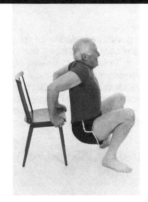

2 *Chair Push-Up:* Face chair seat and stand an arm's length away. Hands grasp front corners of chair seat. Keep legs and body straight while leaning forward enough to feel body weight shift to arms and hands. Now bend elbows and bring knees toward floor, but stop short of touching down. Straighten arms and legs again and repeat this push-up several times.

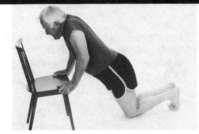

3 *Push-Up and Back Stretch:* Add a long back stretch now. After each push-up, make arms long, back flat, and push hips far back to stretch muscles in back of body. Alternate push-ups with back stretching several times.

Set #6: Coordination Teasers

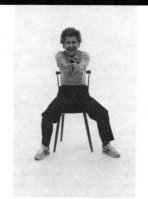 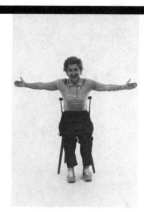

1 **Get Up/Sit Down Confusion:** Sit tall, hands on thighs. Stand up and raise both arms overhead. Sit down and bring hands to thighs. Repeat several times. Now change to sit with arms overhead. Stand up and lower arms. Sit down again and raise arms.

2 **Hand Clap Coordinating:** Sit close to edge of chair. Legs open and close while arms open and close with a hand clap at chest level. Maintain a brisk rhythm. Now change to opposite movements: As legs open, hands clap. As legs come together, arms open wide.

Many of us are not lucky enough to have been born with good coordination. In addition, coordination deteriorates and reaction time slows with aging. However, testing of middle-aged and older persons shows that those who stay physically involved in activities and sports maintain far better coordination and reaction time into the older years than their sedentary contemporaries. The "use it or lose it" principle is at work again here, and these suggested coordination teasers, along with being good exercise, will help to make improvements. Improved coordination and reaction time are important for safety and can help prevent missteps and accidents.

Suggested activities should not bring anyone to the point of frustration. Don't dwell on perfection. Teaching with a sense of humor will help everyone have fun. To avoid making these activities seem like kindergarten games, discuss relevance and purpose: The brain is being challenged to send the right signals quickly to the muscles involved, and repeated practice will result in improvements.

Set #7: Hands and Wrists, Strength and Flexibility

1 **Squeeze and Stretch:** Make tight fists, then stretch fingers as far apart as possible. Start with slow, deliberate movements; then increase speed for nimble fingers. Think of patterns for coordination (e.g., 4 fast/2 slow), counting aloud. These are helpful exercises for arthritic fingers.

2 **Finger Stretch:** With fingers apart, place all fingertips together. Keeping fingers straight and elbows out, gently press fingertips together with little bounces.

3 **Piano Player:** Pretend you are playing a piano, moving all fingers vigorously from side to side.

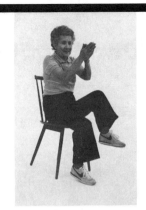 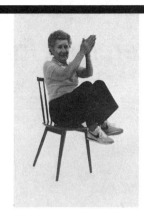

3 *Coordinated Arm Lifting:* Hold hands. Raise and lower arms while legs open and close, touching hands to thighs when legs come together. Opposites come next.

4 *Snap and Stretch Coordination:* Sit tall. Push elbows back at shoulder level, then relax; open arms wide, then bring hands together in front. This pattern is four counts long, legs opening and closing twice. Teach pattern slowly; then increase pace and watch the change to confusion and individual sorting out of movements.

5 *Hand Clap March:* Sit tall and march in place at a brisk pace. Add the three following movements: (a) Clap hands for each knee lift, (b) clap hands on every other knee lift, or (c) lift both knees and clap. Create more patterns.

Cont.

4 *Back Scratcher:* With an imaginary back in front of you, pretend you are vigorously scratching a back, involving finger joints as much as possible.

5 *Wrist Circling:* Lower arms to sides. Moving wrists only, describe circles with hands. Move from inside out a number of times; then change direction.

6 *Hand Warmer:* Rub palms together vigorously to create warmth. Then shake hands out briskly, wrists very loose. For those with poor circulation, this is a quick way to warm cold hands.

exercises for the lower body

Set #8: Leg Strengthening

1   *Weight Shifting:* Stand behind chair, hands on chair back. Legs are more than hip-width apart, toes turned out slightly. Keeping spine erect, shift weight from one leg to the other, bending knee enough to feel quadricep muscles contract.

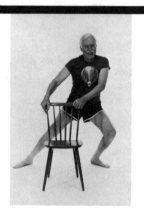

2   *Horseless Rider:* In same leg position, bend knees to a 90° angle, and bounce in this position 10 times before straightening legs to relax. Keep spine erect and hips tucked under. Repeat several times.

5   *Side Leg Lift:* Stand tall, legs together. Raise and lower one leg out to the side as high as it will go without moving upper body. Finish by shaking legs to relax.

6   *Hamstring Stretch:* Place left heel on side edge of chair seat, right hand on chair back. Bend over left leg, keeping it comfortably straight, and let left arm hang. Stay for a short while before changing. Do not bounce in this position.

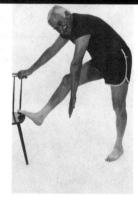

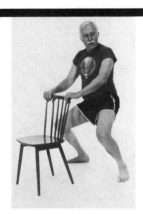

3 ***Half Knee Bends:*** In same leg position, upper body erect, rhythmically bend and straighten legs. Keep pelvis tucked.

4 ***Angle Leg Lift:*** Stand tall, and contract muscles of right leg. Raise and lower leg eight times at an angle to the side of the chair, ball of foot touching lightly each time leg is lowered. Repeat with other leg. Now make the movement more enthusiastic by bending the supporting knee a little and pushing off on each leg lift. Change to raising the knee first, then touching foot to floor, and kicking up at an angle next.

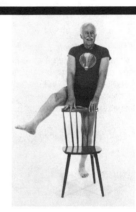

Cont.

Set #9: Foot, Ankle, and Lower Leg Strengthening

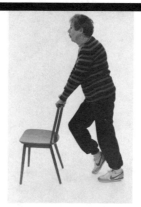 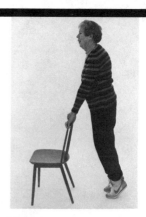

1 *Jog in Place:* Stand behind chair in erect posture, hands on chair back. Roll across soles of feet, raising heel and shifting weight onto ball of foot, rhythmically alternating feet. Get a feeling of having springs under your feet.

2 *Basic Toe Raise:* With feet together, toes pointing straight ahead, raise and lower both heels rhythmically to strengthen feet, ankles, and calves.

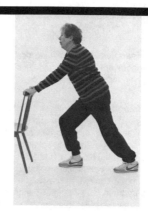

Calf and Heel Cord Stretch: Stretch tired muscles by taking one step back with right leg, heel down and toes pointing straight ahead. Bend left knee toward chair until there is a noticeable stretch in right calf. Stay in this stretch without bouncing. Then change.

Set #10: Low Back Limbering, Buttock Strengthening

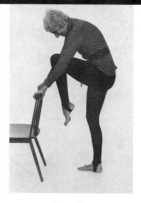 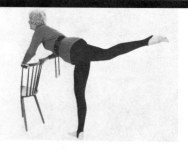

1 *Knee to Nose:* Stand behind chair, hands on chair back. Bring right knee toward nose, rounding spine. Then extend leg straight back and look up. Repeat several times before changing. Now change the angle, bringing knee toward opposite shoulder, then extending leg catty-cornered behind you.

3 *Pigeon-Toed Toe Raise:* With toes turned in, heels apart, raise and lower heels. In this foot position, most demand is placed on outside of feet, ankles, and lower legs.

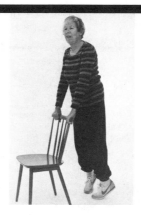

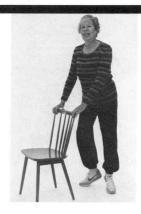

4 *Turned-Out Toe Raise:* Keep heels together, toes turned out. Continue raising and lowering heels to use muscles on inside of lower legs.

Cont.

2 *Back Leg Lift:* Stand erect with chin up. Raise and lower one straight leg directly behind you, feeling buttock muscles contract. This is a small lifting movement, the leg coming only about 1 ft up from floor.

3 *High Leg Lift:* Stand farther away, upper body leaning forward a little. Raise straight leg behind you to hip level, keeping chin up, and return foot to floor. This is a lifting, not a swinging, movement, the buttock muscles contracting on each lift.

4 *Leg Circling:* Stay very erect, chin up. Raise right foot away from floor and draw circles behind you with right leg, from the outside in. Focus on pushing the leg back each time for strong contractions of buttock muscles.

5 Finish by holding chair back with left hand while drawing right knee toward chest with right hand to stretch buttock muscles. Change legs.

Set #11: Standing to Stretch With Chair Support

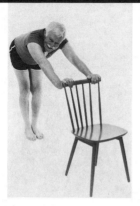

2 *Calf Stretch:* Maintain this position, but stand on heels and pull toes up while pushing hips far back.

3 *Straddle Stretch:* Repeat both stretches with legs apart now.

1 *Long Back Stretch:* Hold chair back and step far enough away to have arms long and back flat. Push hips far back and hold, gently bouncing chest down. Keep head up.

Set #12: Thigh, Hip Flexor, and Abdominal Strength

1 *Double Knee Lift:* Sit close to edge of chair, arms wrapped around chair back, upper back supported. Contract abdominals to maintain rounded back. Bring both knees close to chest; then lower feet to touch floor lightly.

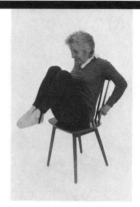

2 *Knee Lift Progression:* In same position, bring knees to chest. Now extend legs up at an angle, toes in line with eyes. Bend knees into chest again; then lower feet to floor. Abdominals must stay contracted throughout to protect lower back. Those who find this exercise too difficult can extend one leg at a time, alternating legs.

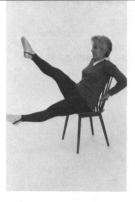

5 *Criss-Crossing Scissor Kick:* Extend both straight legs forward at hip level. Open and cross legs at this level; focus on contracting abdominals to prevent back arching. This exercise becomes easier if legs are lowered a little.

6 Relax tired muscles by sitting back in chair with legs apart. Raise arms into a wide V to inhale deeply. Drop upper body and arms toward floor, relax, and exhale. Repeat several times.

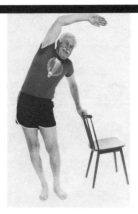

4 ***Side Bending:*** Stand with left hip facing
chair, and place left hand on chair back.
Raise right arm high and bend toward chair,
arm straight and close to ear. Bend left
knee a little, and push hip out to increase
stretch. Repeat on the other side.

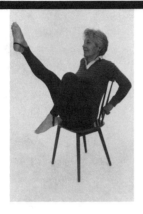

3 ***Bicycle:*** Maintain body position. Perform a
biking motion, starting low and slowly raising legs a little higher. Work at full extension of each leg, and point toes.

4 ***Up/Down Scissor Kick:*** Still sitting at edge
of chair, extend both legs forward, heels on
floor. Keep legs straight while one moves
up, the other down, in rhythmical scissoring.
Do not hold breath. This is a demanding
movement, and those with weak abdominals
should sit back to watch.

Cont.

Set #13: Abdominal and Hip Flexor Strengthening

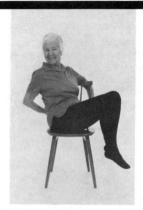

1 *Legs Open and Close:* Sit tall and close to edge of chair, hands grasping sides of chair seat. Lift thighs completely away from chair to bring legs apart. Feet touch floor lightly. Raise thighs again and bring legs together.

2 *Double Leg Swing:* In same position, grasp chair firmly. Legs are together, feet on floor. Lift thighs away from chair and swing both legs to the right, touching feet lightly to floor. Lift again and bring legs far over to the left as hips scoot across chair seat. Pretend that feet have to clear an obstacle on the floor each time legs lift.

Set #14: Leg Strength

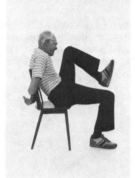
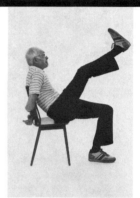

1 *High Leg Extension:* Sit at edge of chair, lean back, and wrap arms around chair back. Bring right knee toward chest, extend leg as high as possible, and lower straight leg to floor. Repeat several times before changing legs.

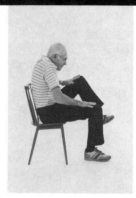

4 *Leg Circling:* Straighten right leg and point toes. Describe circles, starting small and increasing circle size. Alternate legs; then reverse circle direction.

5 *Knee Lift Against Resistance:* Sit up straight and close to edge of chair, palms on thighs. Raise one knee while pushing down against thigh, providing resistance. Alternate legs. This feels as if feet are stuck in mud. Shake legs out.

3 *Progression:* Lift and swing legs to the right, knees bent. Toes touch floor lightly. Now raise and lower knees twice at the right before swinging legs across to the left. The pattern is swing right, lift, lift and swing left, lift, lift. Shake legs out.

2 *Straight Leg Lift:* Straighten right leg out just above floor. Raise and lower straight leg 8 times, keeping quadricep muscles contracted. Lift high each time, and don't quite touch floor on lowering. Change legs.

3 *Toes to Hands:* Stretch arms out at shoulder level. Kick one leg up while bringing arms forward, and touch foot to hands. Open arms wide as foot returns to floor. Kick other leg next, and alternate 10 times.

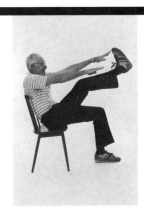

Cont.

Set #15: Legs, Feet, and Fun

1 Stand behind chair for easy jogging in place.

2 Prance around to front of chair and sit down.

3 Quickly get up, prance around chair the other way, and sit down again.

4 Very quickly get up and sit down several times.

5 Stand up, lifting arms overhead to stretch, and sit down again. Repeat several times.

6 Stand up, and *almost* sit down, keeping buttocks just above chair seat. Repeat several times.

Set #16: Chair Polka (Find a happy polka beat for this chair workout.)

1 Sit and briskly tap toes to floor while slapping thighs.

2 Continue toe tapping with hand clapping.

3 Alternate slapping with hand clapping while toe tapping.

4 Lift right knee twice, left knee twice, and continue to change.

5 Slide feet apart and back together with quick heel/toe sliding movements along floor.

6 Touch heel, then toes to floor. Alternate, working with one foot at a time. While flexing and pointing, move foot out to side and back in.

7 Sit down, kick right lower leg forward several times with vigor, and then kick left leg.

8 Sit at edge of chair, lean back, gripping sides of chair seat, and kick both lower legs up a number of times.

9 Prance around to back of chair, hands on chair back, for 10 half knee bends with feet together. Then prance to front of chair and sit down for well-deserved rest.

7 Raise straight right leg. Bend knee out and place ankle on left thigh. Extend leg forward again. Bend the knee and return foot to floor. Alternate legs, keeping a brisk pace to this count of 4.

8 Sit close to edge of chair and lean back. One leg straightens forward, other knee bent. Tap heel of forward foot to floor twice while toes of other foot tap. Change leg position and continue toe and heel tapping. Then change, both legs straightening and bending simultaneously now.

9 Finish with marching in place, clapping hands.

Stretching and Bending Exercises

Set #17: Stretching and Bending

1 **Side Bending:** Sit with legs far apart, feet flat on floor, hips back. Raise left arm, bring it close to ear, and bend to the right, keeping right hand on right thigh for support. Slowly return to upright position and bend to the left.

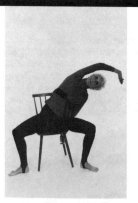

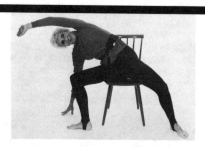

3 **Progression:** Slowly bend to the right and bring right fingertips to floor. Raise left arm as above for a stronger stretch of rib cage, waistline, and outer hip. Slowly come up, and change.

2 **Progression:** Right hand grasps right rear chair leg. With left arm overhead, let right hand slide closer to floor along chair leg. Return to upright position slowly, before changing.

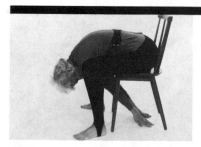

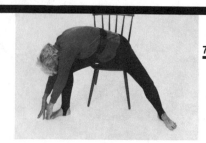

7 **Trunk Circling:** With thumbs still hooked, draw a large circle in the air, moving upper body and arms to the right, down along floor, and up from the left. Circle slowly to prevent dizziness, and change direction after three circles.

Bend and Reach: Continue the above movements, but increase back stretch by reaching through chair legs.

6 **Alternate Reach and Bend:** With arms overhead and thumbs hooked, stretch very tall. Then bend over right leg and touch hands to right foot. Return to tall position, and bend over left leg.

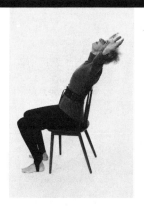 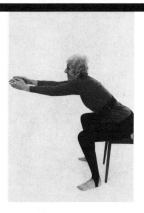 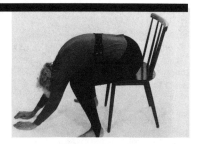

upper body. Hands touch floor, back is round, and head hangs while exhaling.

4 ***Forward Bending:*** Begin in same sitting position, hips back in chair for safety. Raise arms into a wide V, pressing upper back against chair back and arching lower back slightly. Push arms back, look up, and inhale deeply. Now bend forward at waist, arms reaching straight ahead for a long back stretch, chin up. Next, relax arms and

Cont.

Set #18: Twisting and Stretching

1 *Trunk Twisting:* With legs well apart, extend arms out at shoulder level. Keep hips stationary and twist upper body, looking over shoulder. Move slowly.

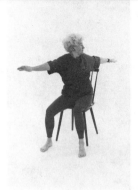

2 *Bent Elbow Twist:* Continue this movement with elbows bent at shoulder level, hands on shoulders. Bounce twice with each twist, pushing elbow back a little farther on second bounce.

Set #19: More Bending, Stretching, Twisting

1 *Shoulder Hold Side Bending:* Begin with hands on shoulders, legs well apart, feet firmly on floor. Slowly bend from side to side, raising one elbow high.

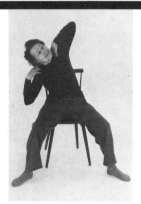

2 *Single Arm Fling:* Sit with back against chair back, legs apart. Elbows are bent at shoulder level, hands at chest. Fling right arm wide, and look at hand as it goes back. Return hand to chest and fling left arm wide.

Set #20: Stretching and Bending

1 *Tall Stretch:* Raise arms overhead. Look up and stretch one arm toward ceiling, bending other elbow. Work at lifting rib cage, stretching waist. Alternate arms rhythmically and comfortably.

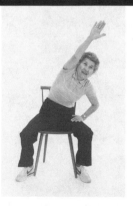
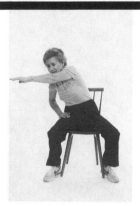

2 *Angle Stretch:* With left hand on thigh, bring right arm across face, reaching toward ceiling at an angle. Stretch arm long and point fingers. Bounce twice; then reach across with left arm.

3 *Crossover Stretch:* Change to reach across chest toward other end of room, upper body following arm.

3 *Tall Stretch:* Lift arms overhead. Hold hands, palms facing ceiling. Straighten arms until upper arms touch ears. Push palms up, feeling a strong stretch in waist and rib cage, and inhale. Lower arms and exhale. Repeat several times.

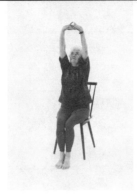

4 *Chest Stretch:* Open arms into a wide V, and press upper back against chair back. Look up and bounce arms back several times. Lower arms to relax. Repeat.

5 *Chest Stretch:* Open arms wide and brace upper back against chair back. Next, cross arms in front of chest. Open and cross arms at shoulder level.

3 *Double Arm Trunk Twisting:* Extend arms forward and hook thumbs. Pull arms from side to side, following movement with head and upper body. Keep arms straight and at shoulder level.

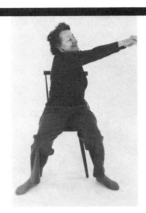

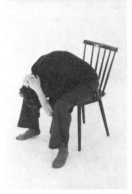

4 *Spine Stretch:* Sit with hands behind neck, legs apart. Slowly bend forward, and try to touch elbows to knees.

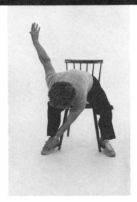

5 *Forward Reaching:* Stay bent forward and stretch both arms straight ahead. Back is flat and long, and one arm at a time reaches forward. Drop arms and upper body, hanging very loosely.

There must be many more ideas to add to these. Develop your own list of chair exercises to keep potentially boring routines challenging, fun, and stimulating. Change is an important spice in keeping exercise interesting and enjoyable.

4 *Crossover Toe Touch:* With legs well apart, bend forward at waist, touching right hand to left foot while left arm lifts high. Then touch left hand to right foot.

9
uplifting ways to end a class

The general mood of the class determines how you spend the last few minutes together. If exercises and activities were well balanced, everyone feels pleasantly tired now and is ready to wind down. The way you end your class sends participants home either bouncy and singing or relaxed and mellow. With sensitivity and awareness, you will know which atmosphere to create at any given time. No matter what you do, the purpose is to create a special feeling of closeness by bringing everyone together after an active hour. Just as it is important to start each class on an up note to encourage enthusiastic participation, make the last few minutes special and harmonious so that everyone feels good about being part of your class. Physical contact with each other supports this good feeling of belonging. Sharing a few quiet minutes of relaxation leaves everyone in a gentle mood, and the good-byes are often accompanied by hugs expressing affection for each other. Choose your music with care for this special time. Let it be something soothing, a gentle, familiar melody everyone (even those who can't carry a tune) wants to hum along with. This, too, creates a good feeling of closeness.

Spend a little time thinking about how you would like everyone to feel as they leave, and then make it happen. Take the time to stay after class, saying good-bye to individuals and sharing a few more unrushed minutes. These are the little thoughtful things that matter so much in making your program and relationships special.

group and relaxation exercises

Set #1: Standing, Circle

If all participants are on their feet toward the end of class, have them come together in a circle and place their hands on each other's upper arms to connect.

1 *Senior Rockettes:* All bring right knee toward chest, return foot to floor, and then kick right leg forward to waist level. Alternate legs to create a reasonably paced rhythm everyone can stay with. Kick with enthusiasm.

2 *Crossover Kick:* Continue this basic pattern, but bring knee across toward other shoulder, then kick leg across. Work together, coordinating knee lifting and kicking to avoid bruises.

Set #2: Standing, Circle

1 *Group Arm Circling:* Stand in circle, legs together, arms wide at shoulder level. Hold hands. Circle all arms from front to back 10 times, then back to front 10 times.

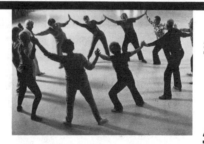

2 *Torso Shift:* With legs apart, extend arms out at shoulder level, palms touching. Moving rib cage only, shift torso to the right, then to the left, pushing against each other's hands.

3 *Weight Shift:* With legs apart and toes turned out slightly, hold each other's upper arms. All right knees bend, shifting weight to the right thigh. Bounce twice, shift weight to the left thigh, and bounce twice. Keep upper body erect, and work together.

4 *Calf Stretch:* Legs together, hands on each other's upper arms. Take one step forward with right leg, chest leading. Keep straight left leg behind you, heel down and toes pointing straight ahead. Bend right knee to create a stretch in the left calf. Stay in this position without bouncing. Bring feet together, and step forward with left leg.

3 *Forward/Back Leg Swing:* All swing the right leg forward, then back, starting low, then increasing height of swing. This becomes an energetic movement, but everyone is stable and balanced by holding on to each other.

4 *Group Bend and Stretch:* Finish by holding hands. Lift arms high, bend back a little, and inhale deeply. Now bend forward, hands toward floor, and bend knees. Exhale loudly to release stress. On each bend, stress is released with greater force, and the noise level becomes quite impressive.

5 *Back Massage:* All make 1/4 turn to the right. Move very close together, one behind the other in the circle, and sit down with legs apart. Scoot around until there is a tight sitting circle, legs on either side of the person's hips in front. Everyone gets busy now massaging shoulders and giving back rubs, receiving a massage at the same time. Use fists for gentle pounding of large back muscles, knead shoulders, and scratch each other's backs. When everyone is warm, place hands on each other's shoulders and slowly lean back to lie down, head coming to rest on a soft body. Relax and feel comfortable resting on this warm padding. To bring the whole group to a sitting position again, push against the shoulders you are holding.

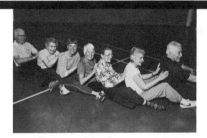
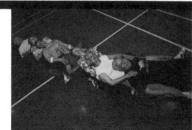

Set #3: Standing, Circle

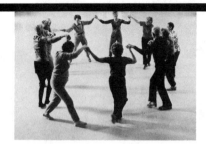

1 *Grapevine Circle:* Hold hands at shoulder level and walk together in the grapevine pattern to the right. Keep knees relaxed and move gracefully, hips swiveling. Repeat, walking to the left.

2 *Coordination Walk:* All hold hands and face right to practice this walking pattern:
a) Starting with the right leg, take 7 long steps to the right. The 8th step is a little swivel jump to change direction for 7 walking steps to the left. Take the 8th step to turn right again.
b) Now break this count of 8 into two sets of 4 steps. Walk 3 steps to the right, swivel on 4, walk 3 steps to the left, swivel, and repeat once more both ways.

Set #4: Partners, Standing

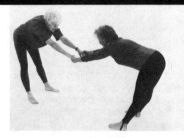 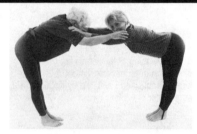

1 *Long Back Stretch:* Hold hands and step away from each other. Legs are together and straight. Help each other stretch arms, shoulders, back muscles, and legs by pushing hips far back.

2 *Straddle Stretch:* Do the same stretch, but stand with legs apart. Bring chest lower.

3 *Shoulder Hold Stretch:* With legs together, put your hands on each other's shoulders. Bend forward at waist, step away from each other, and push gently against partner's shoulders. Back is flat, chin up.

6 *Variation:* Stand side by side, legs apart, inside feet braced. Face same direction, and hold inside hands. Bring outside arms up and hold hands overhead. Both bend the outside knee and pull away from each other. Straighten legs and turn around to stretch again.

7 Combine some of these movements: Start with the Long Back Stretch, then the Shoulder Hold, the Side Bending, Chest Stretch next, and finish with Shoulder Hold.

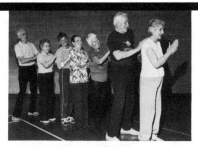

c) Now do four sets of swivel steps only. Keeping legs hip-width apart, swivel on balls of feet, pelvis turning right and left in place, with a little extra bounce to each swivel.

   Count this pattern out loud several times as you practice. When everyone seems to have caught on, walk silently. Start the group off with a loud "1!" as you begin to walk to the right, and then everyone counts quietly and concentrates on staying with the pattern.

3 ***Making Sunshine:*** Stand very close together in the circle and make 1/4 turn to the right. Keep the circle tight, and spend a minute rubbing palms together to create warmth, or "sunshine," that is then rubbed into the upper back and shoulders of the person in front. A happy class ending on a dreary day.

4 ***Chest Stretch:*** Stand back to back and hold hands. Left heels touch. Both step forward with right foot. Bend right knee and pull away from each other, arms straightening behind back. Chest leads, chin points straight ahead. Hold to stretch arms, shoulders, chest, and left lower leg. Change leg position.

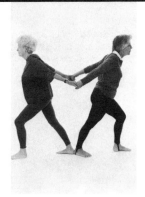

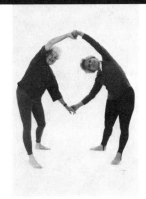

5 ***Side Bending:*** Stand facing each other, legs apart, and hold hands. Bend from side to side comfortably, lifting one set of arms overhead, touching other hands to outside of lower leg.

Cont.

Set #5: Sitting, Facing Each Other

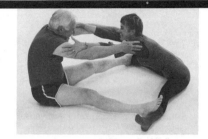

1 *Curl Up and Stretch:* Sit facing each other, legs straight and together. Stretch arms forward, fingertips touching. Now tuck chin close to chest, place hands on legs, and slowly curl spine to floor. Try curling up and reach out for each other again. Repeat several times.

2 *Sit Up and Hug:* With legs apart, reach forward with long arms and try to hug each other, placing hands on each other's upper arms or shoulders. Then, with arms extended forward, slowly curl spine to floor and lie down. Try to curl up again, arms leading, and reach out for another hug.

Set #7: Front-Lying Circle

1 *Torso Lift:* In prone position, all face center of circle and hold hands with arms out at shoulder level. Raise head, arms, and upper body slowly. Return to floor slowly, and repeat twice more.

2 *Long Body Stretch:* With arms stretched straight ahead, work at stretching long, feet pushing away and fingers reaching forward along floor.

3 *Push-Up and Back Stretch:* Place hands next to chest. Moving as a group, everyone straightens arms to raise upper body away from floor. Inhale and look up to stretch abdominals and chest while contracting buttock muscles to avoid hyperextending lower back. Next, push hips back to touch heels, stretching arms and spine, and exhale. Now place arms along body and curl up in the fetal position to relax.

2 *Chest Stretch:* Legs crossed and fingertips on floor directly behind hips. Straighten spine, push shoulders back, and look up while inhaling. Then slump forward, rounding spine, and exhale.

3 *Side Bend:* Legs crossed, right hand on floor next to hip. Raise left arm out and overhead, inhaling, and bend to the right. Increase stretch by sliding right hand away from body. Lower arm while exhaling; then stretch to the left. Repeat several times with deep, relaxed breathing.

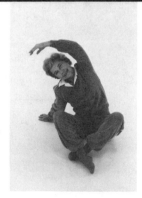

Set #6: Sitting, Circle

1 *Bend and Stretch:* Sit in circle, legs straight and together, and hold hands. All arms lift high. Look up and inhale deeply. Then bend forward, arms stretched long, and exhale forcefully. Repeat several times.

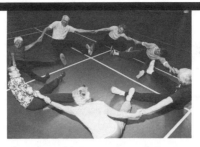

2 *Group Pull:* With legs apart and feet touching, hold hands. Pull to the right, upper body following. Sit up straight again, and pull to the left. Stop short of toppling over.

3 *Leg Crossover:* On back with arms out at shoulder level, hold each other's hands to stabilize upper body. Raise all right legs straight up and inhale. Cross legs over to the left, big toe to floor, and exhale. Raise leg high again, and inhale. Point heel toward ceiling to stretch calf, and slowly return leg to starting position, exhaling. Repeat twice more with same leg; then change for three more crossovers with left leg.

4 *Knee Drops:* Still holding hands, bend knees with feet together on floor. All knees push toward floor at right, heads turning to the left for balance. Inhale as knees come up again; exhale as they lower to the left.

Set #8: Individual Relaxation in Circle

1 *Spine Stretch:* Sit with legs crossed and wrap hands around knees. Pulling firmly against knees, straighten spine, push shoulders back, and inhale deeply. Now lean back to straighten arms, rounding upper back, chin close to chest, while exhaling. Repeat several times.

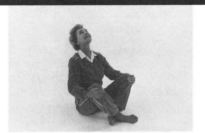

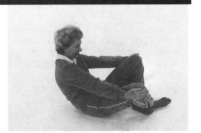

Cont.

4 *Arm Raising:* Sit with legs crossed and raise both arms out and overhead where hands meet, inhaling deeply. Then bend forward, touching hands to floor, and exhale. Raise arms overhead, sit erect, and inhale. Lower arms out and down to starting position while exhaling.

Set #9: Head Movements

1 Sit tall, legs crossed, hands around knees. Raise head, point chin up, and inhale. Then bring chin toward chest and exhale. Repeat slowly several times.

2 Turn head to the right, looking over right shoulder. Slowly turn head to the left and look over left shoulder.

3 Sit tall. Tilt head, bringing right ear toward right shoulder; then tilt head slowly toward left shoulder.

4 With chin close to chest and spine very straight, swing head like a pendulum, stretching back of neck.

5 Straighten legs and shake them out to relax.

Set #11: Chair-Sitting Relaxation

For some, sitting on the floor is not comfortable enough for true relaxation. They may find sitting on chairs more conducive to letting go and feeling limp. Move into a circle, joining each other for the last few minutes of class. Combine all movements with deep, relaxed breathing.

1 *Upper Back, Arm, and Finger Stretch:* Clasp hands and inhale deeply. Push arms forward at shoulder level, palms facing away. Lean forward slightly, stretch arms long, and exhale. Sit up again, bringing hands to chest, and repeat several times.

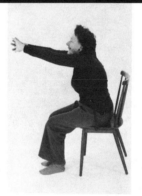

2 *Stretch Forward and Up:* Push palms straight ahead again, leaning forward. Then raise arms overhead, palms toward ceiling, and stretch very tall. Relax, lowering hands to thighs, and repeat several times.

3 *Head Press:* Sit tall, hands clasped behind head. Press head against hands, simultaneously pressing hands against head, elbows open, and inhale. Exhale, rounding upper back and bringing elbows forward.

5 *Single Arm Stretch:* Sit erectly, hands at shoulders, palms up. Slowly straighten right arm, palm toward ceiling, and really stretch tall. Look up and inhale. Return hand to shoulder and exhale. Repeat with left arm, lifting rib cage and feeling trim.

6 *Double Arm Raising:* Sit tall, arms down and relaxed. Raise arms out and overhead, inhaling deeply, and bring hands together. Work at stretching very tall. Lower arms to sides while exhaling, and repeat several times.

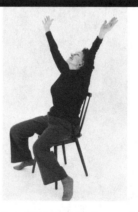

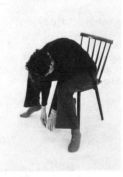

7 *Stretch and Drop:* Sit with legs apart, hips back. Raise arms into a wide V, stretch, and inhale. Then bend forward, back round and relaxed, arms and head hanging. Touch hands to floor and exhale. Repeat several times. To finish, stay in forward position, upper body and arms very relaxed, top of head pointing at floor. Blood and oxygen is brought to the head; come up slowly to prevent dizziness.

Set #10: Back-Lying Relaxation, Muscles Contract and Relax

1 Relax arms. Contract buttocks strongly, hold contraction for a few seconds, and relax.

2 Contract abdominals and thighs, hold, and relax.

3 Make tight fists, contract arm muscles, hold, and relax.

4 Push heels away, stretching calves, hold, and relax.

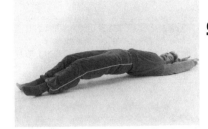

5 With arms overhead, contract buttocks, abdominals, and thighs. Raise hips away from floor. Hold for a few seconds; then relax whole body.

6 Again, contract all large muscle groups and raise body away from floor. Keep contact with heels, shoulder blades, head, and arms only. Arch up, feeling very tight. Then relax completely. Take a deep breath and stretch, then curl up with knees to chest, arms wrapped around knees, and exhale.

4 *Self-Hug:* Sit back in chair, upper back against chair back. Open arms wide at shoulder level, and inhale deeply. Now hug yourself, wrapping hands around shoulders. Upper back is round and head hangs forward as you exhale.

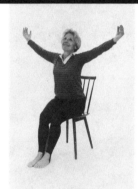 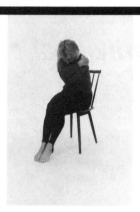

Cont.

Set #12: Self-Massage

A self-massage is a real treat, something we usually don't bother making time for, but it's a wonderful way to relax and feel better in just a few minutes. Include it occasionally at the end of a class; it's a nice way to get in touch with yourself.

1   **Shoulder Massage:** Place right hand on left shoulder to knead muscles. Kneading improves blood circulation and releases muscle tension, and it's good exercise for arthritic hands. After kneading, rub up and down firmly between neck and shoulder, fingers pointing behind you, to create friction and warmth. Don't forget the other shoulder.

2   **Neck Massage:** Place all fingertips on back of neck. With small circular motions, press fingertips into neck muscles, moving up to base of skull and back down into shoulder muscles. Continue this gentle digging till hands are tired. Shake them out to relax.

3   **Neck Rub:** Place open palms to back of neck. Rub neck and shoulders firmly, using fingers and palms.

4   **Bone Massage:** Place tips of middle and forefingers on bone behind ears. Firmly massage up and down along this bone.

5   **Nose and Eye Massage:** Place thumbs on jaw bones, middle and forefingers on bridge of nose. Massage nose gently with fingertips. Move thumbs to cheek bones. Gently place fingertips on closed eye lids. Very gently massage eyes, stroking from nose toward cheek bones only. Then massage bony protrusion above eyes, again stroking from nose outward.

6   **Forehead Massage:** Put thumbs on cheek bones near ears, middle and forefingers meeting at center of forehead. With fingertips, stroke firmly from center of forehead out, following line of eyebrows. Don't apply pressure over temples.

individual exercise advice

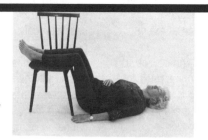

7 *Face Massage:* Put all fingertips along nose and cheek bones with firm pressure, stroking from nose to sides of face only. Then place palms to cheeks and rub in small circular movements.

All massaging and rubbing increases blood circulation, creates warmth through friction, and melts away muscle tension and tiredness.

8 Finish in *the most comfortable position in the world*: Rest on your back and place lower legs sideways across chair seat as shown. To be very comfortable, place a sweatshirt or sweater under your head. Rest arms along body, hands open and loose. The spine should be in good alignment, knees directly above hips, and lower legs relaxed on chair seat. Close your eyes and breathe deeply and slowly. Stay for a minute or two, and let yourself go limp.

Use of chronological age cannot be a measuring stick for function and ability. We find great individual differences as we observe any group of people, and this is certainly true of those over 60. Just look at your older students: Some are thin, some overweight. Some are energetic and strong, some frail and slow. Some stand and walk tall and proud; others are stooped and take cautious steps. Many are in good health, others have physical limitations. All these and many more variations need to be appreciated to understand and accept that there should be many levels of participation within a group. We encourage participants to monitor themselves and work around individual limitations to make group exercise safe and comfortable for all. In addition, we can be helpful and supportive when individuals come to us for personal exercise advice.

Individual concerns and questions require a reliable combination of good judgment and common sense and a knowledge of the person's health status and present level of physical condition. By staying alert throughout each class, you will quickly become aware of those who seem to have a problem, and a personal conversation is the first step in exploring what may be wrong. When you feel in the least uncertain about your ability to give sound advice, suggest that the participant call or visit a doctor's office first and report back to you. Some of the most common conditions we are likely to encounter among participants in our programs are discussed in the medical chapter. This, in addition to personal contacts with physicians when necessary, should provide a helpful basis for individual exercise advice. In addition, there is basic commonsense advice to be shared with everyone:

1. If you have been very sedentary, a medical exam helps remove apprehensions and supports your desire to improve your physical condition.
2. Exercise needs to be adapted to your present condition and health status. If exercise is too easy, it brings little benefit and improvement, and if it's too strenuous, you will feel discouraged and unwell.
3. Exercise should be progressive. Start at a comfortable level, build up slowly, and improve to participate more vigorously and for longer periods of time.
4. Exercise should not be occasional and sporadic; a commitment to regular participation is important for good health.
5. Whatever form of activity you choose, let it be a positive experience. Your mental attitude will determine the physical benefits you derive.
6. Adjust your level of exercise to heat and humidity, which place stress on the cardiovascular system.
7. Always slow down if you feel fatigued or find yourself short of breath.
8. Stop if you feel dizzy or nauseous.
9. Heart palpitations or abnormal heart rhythms need to be checked by your physician.
10. Don't exercise if you are sick, especially if you have a fever.
11. Don't compete with anyone else. You are not training for the Olympics. Trust the good judgment you have developed over many years of living. Slow down or stop, even if everyone else keeps going.
12. Eliminate all exercises that cause pain or discomfort, unless you have a diagnosed condition that precludes painfree movement.

These basic precautions should not be hurdles or limits but are sensible guidelines for safe and health-promoting exercise. They apply to everyone at every age.

Newton's first law of dynamics says, "An object at rest tends to stay at rest," and this certainly applies to people. Finding excuses for not exercising is common at every age if the person is not naturally inclined to exercise. People are too busy, too tired, too overworked, have aches and pains. The list is long, but it can be quickly shortened with your encouragement. Many older people believe that their need for exercise diminishes and eventually disappears as they get older. There is a tendency to exaggerate the risks of exercise and to overrate the benefits of light, sporadic exercise. Activities like light housework, bowling, golf with electric carts, or window shopping tend to be considered adequate for maintenance of fitness.

When we meet as a group, we help new participants take the important first step away from a low level of fitness. These two scheduled hours of exercise each week help remove apprehensions and change attitudes. If we encourage participants to build another half hour of individual exercise into each day, the amount of time spent moving can change Newton's statement into a more positive one: "An object in motion tends to stay in motion." Overcoming inertia is the major hurdle. Developing motivation and self-discipline for adherence and additional individual exercise is the next step. With appropriate guidance and support, we can help with this task, too. Shortness of breath, aching backs, poor posture, creaking joints, and low energy levels can be improved if the desire is there. This desire to get rid of the blahs, to want to feel as well as possible, is much more valuable than a prescription for pills and potions.

It is well documented that gains of physical activity are lost with a few weeks of inactivity or bed rest. Consequently, participants must be continually encouraged to keep moving, not only in our classes but in their daily lives. To encourage additional individual exercise, share these basic arguments for improved personal fitness:

prolonged independence

Prolonged independence is a major motivator. Much attention has been focused on increased longevity, but the quality of life, continued independence, and self-sufficiency in the older years may be of greater concern. The average senior citizen spends 5.3 years with a major limitation of daily activity. A number of factors may contribute to such disability, but a major one is muscular decline and weakness due to disuse. There are many reasons that motivate younger persons to exercise. The high-tech approach to exercise is appealing, cosmetic concerns are powerful motivators, and the possible prevention of heart disease is another strong incentive. These reasons for becoming or staying active are largely eliminated at an older age but can be replaced with other, more relevant incentives. Prolonged independence may very well be at the top of the list because no one desires dependent living and need for care.

lifestyle

Lifestyle may be strongly affected by a commitment to regular exercise. An active lifestyle encourages other healthy habits. Many smokers are helped in their efforts to give up this habit once exercise has become a positive part of their lives. Exercise develops body awareness and greater appreciation of overall good health. Consequently, eating habits tend to improve, dieting becomes more effective, and alcohol consumption is reduced. Exercise adds something very positive to the individual's life and makes it easier to modify lifestyle habits that are not health-promoting.

mental attitude

Mental attitude and mood can be strongly influenced by physical activity. The disengagement from social life and other involvements so common at older ages can be turned around, especially through organized group programs. Here, new challenges can be faced and met. Physical self-confidence and self-image improve, new friendships are formed, and there is ready-made cheerful social interaction to counter loneliness and withdrawal. Participation in physical activity may very well be the first step to opening doors to other involvements that will make life more satisfying and meaningful.

overall wellness

Overall wellness and a high energy level are prime motivators for continued activity. Stiffness and minor pains in muscles, joints, and bones can become a reminder to keep moving rather than an excuse to give in and give up. Such pains and discomforts become a familiar part of living as we age, but a positive exercise experience helps us believe that they are in part the result of inactivity and can be minimized. Exercise can be therapy and medical prophylaxis and has value in a wide range of disorders as discussed in the medical chapter. Regular activity results in our feeling better, having more energy, minimizing aches and pains, and feeling in charge. The overall quality of daily life can improve significantly and become the ultimate motivation for staying as active as is reasonably possible.

Be very liberal in your reminders not to let a day slip by without including as much natural exercise as possible.:

* Find reasons to use your stairs at home as many times as possible each day.
* Avoid escalators and elevators. Just pretend they aren't there, and climb a flight or two of stairs instead.
* Park your car several blocks away from where you need to go and walk the rest of the way.
* Get out for a long brisk walk and fresh air daily if at all possible. President Harry Truman walked 1-1/2 miles every morning at a purposeful pace. "If you are going to walk for your physical benefit," he said, "it's necessary that you walk as if you are going someplace!"
* Take a friend for a walk instead of meeting for a caloric lunch.
* Hang your laundry in the breeze instead of using your dryer. You can sneak in some stretching, bending, and lifting.
* Get a long phone cord. Move around if you spend a lot of time on the phone.
* Wash windows, rake leaves, pull weeds. Keep all parts moving at all cost, and don't let others do for you what you can still do yourself.
* Always remember the old fitness saying, "Never lie down when you can sit, never sit when you can stand, and never stand when you can walk." And to this I add, "Never use your car when you can walk, and don't walk slowly if you can walk briskly."

Something participants in my classes have appreciated is a poster of exercises I had printed for use at home. I cannot think of anyone who has not been able to do these basic exercises at home comfortably and safely after I have demonstrated them clearly in the classroom. They are of low intensity and use major muscle groups and joints. I know that my students use this poster faithfully, taking between 10 and 15 minutes in the morning to start their day off right, and you may want to develop something along these lines for your group. I have found that a bright, cheerful poster leaves far more impact than a small handout, which tends to end up in waste baskets. Most of my students have this poster pinned to their bedroom door as a daily reminder to "use it or lose it."

10
the physiology of aging

Those who exercise regularly notice nice results: Scale weight may go down while self-esteem goes up. Muscles tighten and flab disappears. Stamina, strength, and endurance improve along with outlook, and there is an overall feeling of good health and high energy. Exercise physiologists, in their academic course work and laboratories, investigate the "why" of exercise (rather than the "how to," which is the physical educator's concern). They look, for example, at changes in metabolic rate (or energy requirement) during exercise: How many calories are burned with what activity? While test subjects run on a relentlessly moving treadmill, oxygen consumption is measured. Body composition is studied, estimating percent of stored body fat and calculating lean body mass. Stress testing provides important information on how the heart/lung system responds to exercise. Neuromuscular responses are studied with the help of sophisticated digital timers capable of measuring one one-thousandth of a second. The usefulness of exercise science is examined in terms of practical application to, for example, improving athletic performance. Exercise science is a relatively new discipline, but it has made significant contributions to the advancement of knowledge about human performance. But looking at the relationship between exercise and aging has not been a research priority for exercise physiologists, and the paucity of good data, and of programs to prove the value of exercise in later life, is frustrating for those teaching related courses.

available research

Benjamin Ricci, professor of exercise science at the University of Massachusetts, teaches a course entitled "Anatomical and Physiological Aspects of Aging" each fall. "The problem with teaching this course is that there is no rich data base to turn to," says Dr. Ricci. "Researchers—and I have been guilty of this in the past myself—have largely relied on the conveniently available student population for most of their studies and then extrapolated to older people, and that simply does not work. Data which has been collected using older subjects tends to be biased since these studies usually involve master swimmers, runners, or other unusually active persons. The conclusions drawn from looking at these athletic older individuals are ultimately not very useful because these subjects represent just a very small percentage of the older population. Those who volunteer as subjects for such studies tend to be activity-oriented, and it's a little hard to find the variety of subjects needed to arrive at meaningful results which would give us a sound basis for making exercise recommendations for older persons."

Dr. Ricci's special interest in the area of exercise and aging is in part personal. "At 62, I am getting old by all standards. But 62 is just a chronological number. I feel young, and looking at medical indicators and how I score on fitness tests, I am certainly much younger physiologically than chronologically." His most recent blood pressure reading astonished his physician to the point of retaking it several times: 128 over 84 is not typical of a person his age. His blood pressure reading indicates resilient blood vessels, and his stamina, strength, endurance, and energy level are high. And yet, "formal" exercise is not part of Dr. Ricci's life. "I am not fond of structured, regimented exercise, and the exercise equipment most people seem to need to do something physical is not part of my life. But I love physical activity, the normal, everyday use of the body." There is not even a sweatsuit in his wardrobe, and yet he is in fine physical condition. "I don't need a costume to change into. I buy clothes to be functional so that I can put normal activity into every workday."

Despite his extensive knowledge about the whys and hows of exercise, Dr. Ricci's suggestions for staying well and fit are as simple as Grandma's words of wisdom. It's not the kind of advice people are anxiously waiting for, though; there aren't any special gimmicks.

"Walking is great, and a very normal part of my daily life. The car stays home. I get off the bus a distance away from campus and get a good, brisk walk in before work. During the day, my feet take me everywhere on campus—to meetings, classes, and lunch. I probably walk around 5 miles a day and never think of it as 'exercise.' It gets me where I need to go, and I thoroughly enjoy it. At my age, it's not hard to get my heart rate up into the 'target zone' with brisk walking so that it qualifies as aerobic exercise. But you have to move at a good pace." He admits to doing 30 sit-ups, some pull-ups, and push-ups every morning, but he likes to get those over with in short order. "It's just enough stress to keep my muscles toned; beyond that I use normal, everyday activities and physical work to meet my exercise needs."

On his 25 acres of property, there is plenty of exercise in the form of work: He cuts trees and chops four cords of firewood each year, keeps his old farmhouse in shape, cares for a large yard ("No riding lawnmower for me!"), and enjoys walking and hiking on his property. He is an avid birdwatcher and photographer, hobbies that add extra miles of walking.

Dr. Ricci's exercise recommendations for older persons certainly do not include weight training or jogging, the two most popular forms of exercise today. "In midlife, many people expect to recapture youth over a few weeks, and what they get instead is problems and injuries. If I were a professional wrestler, I would need the force, bulk, and muscle mass that weight training has to offer to help me do something effective against my opponent. The same would be true for a football player. But middle-aged or older persons are no longer wrestling or playing football. They need to stay functional instead, to have stamina for everyday demands, to be able to take a long brisk walk with a friend and carry on a conversation without gasping for breath after a few minutes. Everyone, even in the older years, should be able to get through the day without falling apart at 5 o'clock. But the attempt to use the body to displace enormous weights is out of the realm of normal exercise. For many, it becomes ego gratification, just like compulsive running. It has little to do with health."

Dr. Ricci has made a strong commitment to working toward more extensive research into the effects exercise and lifestyle may have on aging. He has an ambitious plan for which he is laying the groundwork now and to which he will devote his retirement: In conjunction with the University of Massachusetts Medical School in Worcester, he intends to develop a large-scale computer inventory, collecting data on how people live and how it affects them as they grow older. "We need to involve people of different age groups in this study, starting with those in their 20s. And by the time these young people have grown old, researchers will get a good picture of how lifestyle and exercise affect aging, and then we will be able to see whether what we now believe really has validity. We will need to find people who are not only willing to participate in this longitudinal study but will also donate their bodies as anatomical gifts for postmortem research."

Dr. Ricci's body has already been donated. "I can give clear information about what my lifestyle has been, and my heart, arteries, lungs, and other organs can be looked at to see whether their condition reflects my lifestyle. Such research has not been done before, but if we want to find answers to the questions we are now asking, we have to make a start. At this time, we are making a lot of assumptions, and it's time to go beyond that. And even though I won't be around to see the results of these long-term studies, I want this work to be my contribution long after I am gone."

A lifestyle of moderation is what Professor Ricci has adhered to, and this, he believes, is the ultimate answer. "We need to keep balance in our lives and stay away from excesses. Excessive eating is just as bad as excessive exercise. There is nothing wrong with enjoying a glass of wine with dinner, but heavy drinking is damaging. The kind of stress and fast pace that's part of today's living undermines our health. By staying active, we can keep better emotional balance in our lives, work off a lot of stress, keep blood pressure down, and sleep well. People try to cram too much into a lifetime; they run faster and harder without getting anywhere. I would very much like to see a strong national wellness movement, for all ages. It's never too late to make improvements in lifestyle, and that message has to get across loud and clear to all of us. We have made a small start, but it's very puzzling to realize that the concept of moderation simply doesn't appeal to the general public. Fads and excesses are likely to continue, which will not improve our national health picture. We need to examine what is driving people so hard because it is frightening."

research and classroom observations

Regular contacts and discussions with Dr. Ricci and others in exercise science have been of great interest and help to me in my work with seniors over the years. It is always satisfying when I find that a conclusion I have drawn from practical experience in the classroom is supported by scientifically conducted studies. I have the privilege of observing the impressive effects regular exercise has on older individuals. My friends in exercise science put their stamp of scientific approval on these observations and agree that their findings support what I see happen over and over again. Priscilla Clarkson, associate professor of exercise science at the university here, put it very simply in a recent conversation: "Some of our research findings are really not terribly surprising, different, or new. We logically know that an active lifestyle promotes better health and physical ability as we get older. We know intuitively that there are certain prerequisites if we want quality in our older years. It is logical that decline can be minimized if regular exercise is continued throughout life. But it is important to confirm these logical assumptions scientifically and to be able to give sound exercise recommendations for older persons based on these findings."

Such research data helps us exercise leaders understand the normal responses of the older person's body to exercise so that we can plan our programs accordingly. An individual's exercise capacity affects almost all aspects of life—not just what can be physically accomplished, but also, and just as importantly, how individuals feel abut themselves and how much enjoyment there is in life at an older age.

"It is not an easy task to separate the effects of aging from what is termed disuse atrophy or lack of exercise," says Vickie Foster, exercise physiologist at the University of Colorado in Boulder. "Many older persons do not recognize that there have been physical changes until performance capability is seriously lowered. And even though these changes occur inevitably with time, they can be tremendously modified by an active lifestyle. Regardless of the government's decision to classify old as being over 65 years of age, we all know people in their 30s who have old minds and bodies. Those of us who have had the privilege of working with older persons in our programs have seen individuals in their 80s and even 90s who maintain a youthful outlook and whose bodies are physiologically much younger than their years. Because of these tremendous individual differences, it is important to classify older exercisers not only according to chronological age, but also with regard to their specific physical capabilities and limitations."

It is an accepted fact that aging causes a number of alterations in the systems of the body. "Lack of movement may be a key factor in many of these alterations," Professor Foster points out, "and it is important to look at how exercise can help to stem the tide of decline. Scientists have documented many of the manifestations of age but have been unable in many cases to determine to what extent we should implicate age, abuse of our bodies, or simply lack of activity. More and more research indicates that we can greatly modify many of the functional and structural changes associated with age by a healthy, active lifestyle. Those of us interested in researching the effects of exercise on aging are ultimately motivated by believing that functional decline can be signficantly slowed if we don't start to take it easy but stay active instead."

I want to thank my friends Priscilla Clarkson, Vickie Foster, and Benjamin Ricci for contributing to this chapter on age-related physiological changes. The information gives basic understanding of how the various body systems respond to exercise and how studies involving older subjects provide insight into changes in these responses with aging. Further informative reading is suggested at the end of this guide.

the cardiorespiratory system and aging

The heart, lungs, and vessels of the circulatory system form the pump and plumbing of the body. This system transports nourishment and oxygen to the tissues of the body where metabolic processes produce energy. The cardiorespiratory system also transports waste products away from the sites of energy production. Healthy function of this system is essential for a healthy life.

When we work or exercise, the working muscles increase their demand for oxygen, and the cardiorespiratory system responds. Some of these exercise effects are familiar to all of us: Demanding exercise makes us breathe harder, and the heart starts to beat faster. As the heart begins to pump more forcefully, the amount of blood pumped with each beat (stroke volume) increases. Increased cardiac output allows the circulatory system to deliver freshly oxygenated blood to the muscles more rapidly so that exercise or work efforts can be sustained.

In meeting the body's demands for more oxygen and efficient removal of metabolic waste products, the work load on the heart is greatly increased. Since the heart itself is a muscle, oxygen must go to the heart cells (myocardium). The heart has its own circulatory system to supply the necessary nutrients and oxygen. Maintenance of healthy coronary arteries, free from blockage by fatty plaques, is one of the important health issues of the modern world. If blockage, usually caused by arteriosclerosis or atherosclerosis, develops, the heart's ability to provide adequate oxygen for strenuous exercise is reduced, and physical output will be limited.

At the working muscles, exercise causes changes in metabolic function. Oxygen is exchanged for carbon dioxide at the small vessels of the circulatory system, the capillaries. During exercise, the muscle cells can increase the amount of oxygen extracted for energy production almost threefold.

The lungs contribute to help meet the muscle's need for the exchange of oxygen and carbon dioxide. It is important that there be fast and efficient exchange if exercise demands are to be met. The total amount of air moved (ventilation) increases because of faster and deeper breaths. The capillaries in the lungs open for greater flow of blood, providing a greater surface area of exchange with the small air sacs in the lungs, the alveoli.

the effects of aging on the cardiorespiratory system

Aging affects the cardiorespiratory system in a number of ways. Maximal heart rate shows a progressive decline starting at about 25 years of age. This decline is estimated to occur at the rate of one beat per year. Studies show, however, that the widely used formula of (220 − age in years) may be low since a maximum heart rate of 170 beats per minute is not unusual for persons in their 60s. Stroke volume as well as cardiac output shows a decrease with aging, most noticeably during hard exercise, at an estimated 10 to 20% compared to a young adult. Although the young person's cardiovascular system easily adapts to increased exercise demands, this same stress may not be tolerated by the older individual due to possible hypertension, malfunction of the heart valves, degeneration of the heart itself, or arterial changes. Warning symptoms include excessive shortness of breath during exercise, anginal pain, poor recovery from exercise, and undue fatigue. If an older person shows these types of symptoms, intensity and duration of the activity must be adjusted accordingly.

If abnormalities are detected during electrocardiographic studies, caution is indicated when prescribing exercise. On the other hand, few senior citizens would participate in activity if those with unusual electrocardiograms were prevented from exercise. If exercise is moderate and sensible, the risk of developing problems has been shown to be very low. According to Dr. Roy Shepard of the Toronto Rehabilitation Center program, the incidence of cardiac emergencies is one for every 110,000 hours of exercise, or one episode in 15 class years for a typical class of 50 participants meeting three times per week. "Everyone working with the elderly should certainly be prepared to undertake two or three resuscitations in the course of his or her career, but such events are not frequent enough to have a major influence upon the decision to exercise," Dr. Shepard concludes. He feels that it is important for participants to know how to take their pulse accurately, to recognize the symptoms of exertional angina, and to hold exercise demands below a level that would cause negative symptoms.

Changes in the elasticity of major blood vessels have been recognized for many years. Blood vessels tend to become more rigid with aging, with narrowing and occasional obstruction of vessels supplying both the heart and the skeletal muscles. Because blood vessels are less elastic, they accept blood pumped by the heart less readily than a younger person's. Increased blood pressure results, and the heart has to work harder not only during exercise but even at rest. The maximum amount of oxygen the muscle cells can extract from the blood also declines. In the older person, this change may be related to a decrease in the saturation level of blood with oxygen, a decrease in hemoglobin (the carrier of oxygen in the blood), and/or a poor distribution of blood to the muscles. Some studies also have shown that older people have a loss of mitochondria in the muscles. These are small organelles in the cells that are primarily responsible for the generation of aerobic energy. Other studies have shown that the enzymes that act as catalysts for many energy production reactions may also decrease with age.

The airways and lungs are subject to lifelong contact with noxious substances contained in the environment, and it is difficult to separate the effects of these environmental factors from age-related functional changes in the respiratory system. After the age of 30, people experience a slow but progressive loss of lung function. Though few longitudinal studies have been conducted, they do indicate a general decline until the sixth decade, followed by a more accelerated loss. These observed changes are difficult to generalize, however, because of the great variations from one individual to the next. But it is known that in advanced age a loss of functional alveoli (air sacs) and associated capillary network occurs, which results in a decrease in the lung surface area available for gas exchange. Lungs become less elastic, and total lung capacity decreases. There is a change in the elasticity of the chest wall, and respiratory muscle strength and elasticity decline, affecting the ability to sustain an increased breathing rate. Lung capacity is also significantly affected by years of smoking. The maximal oxygen intake has declined by about 35% at age 65, and this rate of decline may in part be due to an individual's health history.

exercise and the aging cardiorespiratory system

Although exercise cannot totally reverse these changes associated with age, it can certainly reduce the rate and degree of decline for most people. With exercise, the older person can expect to see a number of training effects similar to those observed in younger individuals. Resting heart rate will be lowered. Stroke volume increases, as does cardiac output. The muscles demonstrate an increased ability to extract oxygen, and the volume of blood in the cardiovascular system increases. Resting blood pressure will generally be lower, and the entire system becomes more efficient in the distribution of blood. Increased breathing capacity and cardiorespiratory efficiency also occur as a result of exercise training. An older individual cannot expect to maintain or achieve the same level of fitness as a trained young person, primarily because of the age-related decline in maximum heart rate. However, the older fit individual will have a considerably greater exercise capacity than a sedentary person at the same age.

The positive cardiorespiratory changes that occur in the older person who participates in a regular exercise program can markedly enhance the ability to cope with the demands of daily living. Exercise provides a reserve capacity that enables the older person to participate in and enjoy life fully.

neuromuscular function

Muscle is mechanical in nature. When muscles contract, chemical energy is converted to mechanical energy. Three types of muscle tissue are found in the body: smooth, cardiac, and skeletal. Smooth muscle contracts automatically and is associated with many of the internal organs. Cardiac muscle is the specialized muscle tissue of the heart. Skeletal muscle comprises approximately 40% of the body mass and makes all movement possible. All muscle tissues require nerve supply for contraction.

A motor neuron, or nerve, together with the muscle fibers it stimulates is called a motor unit. The motor neuron releases a chemical substance to the muscle that causes it to contract. The degree of force exerted by the muscle is controlled by the frequency of stimulation of motor units and the total number of units recruited. Because some motor units are active at one time and others at another, we are able to smoothly coordinate a variety of movements.

There are a number of terms to know when discussing the practical aspects of neuromuscular function. *Muscular strength* is a measure of the maximal force a muscle or set of muscles can exert in a single voluntary contraction. In comparison, *muscular endurance* is achieved by repetitive contractions of a portion of muscle fibers. *Speed of movement* includes both reaction time and movement time. The time it takes from stimulus presentation to the start of movement is termed reaction time. Movement time indicates the amount of time from initial response to the completion of movement. Also of importance is *neuromuscular coordination*, which involves reaction time, movement time, and both fine (small muscle) and gross (large muscle) motor skills.

Many different types of muscular activity can occur with exercise. Weight training is primarily a strength activity, whereas walking and jogging involve muscular endurance. Power is required for activities such as jumping, and neuromuscular coordination is important in sport participation and, of course, in everyday living.

effects of aging
on the neuromuscular system

With age, almost all of these aspects of neuromuscular function decline. Aging causes decrease in strength, muscular endurance, speed of movement, power, and coordination. These measurable changes are associated with a decrease in nerve conduction speed and the number of fibers in a given motor unit. Additionally, the fast-contracting muscle fibers are selectively lost with age. The result is that older muscle takes longer to respond to a neural stimulus. The biochemical profile of the older muscle is also adversely altered with age, resulting in a reduction in muscular performance capabilities.

Professor Priscilla Clarkson, exercise physiologist at the University of Massachusetts, is particularly interested in investigating neuromuscular changes in aging. "On the outside, we can see that an aging person's muscles become 'flabby.' I am involved in looking at what is going on inside the muscle that makes this atrophy happen. Are the muscle fibers getting smaller, or are they disappearing? And it seems that with aging both these things happen: There is a decrease in number of fibers as well as in size."

The study Clarkson conducted several years ago involved subjects between the ages of 65 and 70. "We took small biopsy samples of muscle tissue and found that it was the fast twitch (strength) fibers in the muscle which were decreasing most in size. So we believe that lack of use causes these fibers to degenerate and results in the muscle atrophy we see in aging. And this presents a new picture in the exercise physiology world. We already have a body of literature indicating that the incidence of heart attacks increases with age. Everyone knows that exercise and a generally healthy lifestyle helps decrease a person's risk for heart disease and heart attack. As a result, exercise physiologists have given their recommendations for aerobic exercise such as walking, jogging, or swimming. But the muscle physiologist tells the aging person that it is important to add some type of strength and muscle toning program to this aerobic activity to maintain the strength fibers and reduce muscle atrophy. It has been shown that hypertrophy (enlargement) can be induced in older muscles. The type of strength activities we would generally suggest for older persons would not cause a large amount of hypertrophy but would increase muscle tone and maintain adequate strength."

Clarkson's study looked at a group of sedentary folks and compared them to a group whose lifestyle had been and continued to be active. "There was a great difference in fast twitch fiber size between the active and inactive subjects, despite the fact that aging inflicts

atrophy even on the active person. Muscle atrophy simply is a normal part of aging—but we find in our studies that the active older individual's losses are very different from what the inactive person experiences. The active group we studied scored about halfway between young subjects and the 'old inactives'—not a bad place to be considering that general physical demands do decrease as we get older. And we weren't even looking at exercisers but at people who lived an active, normal life. When we did these studies about 6 years ago, there was little general interest in weight training—that is a recent development. It would be very interesting to look at these muscle changes if a person were to participate in a weight-training program into older age. I assume losses would be even smaller."

Both animal and human data indicate that degeneration takes place not only in the muscle fibers but also in the nerve that attaches to these fibers. "Something more central is degenerating, and it shows up in the muscle fibers." By having subjects respond to a reactor light with a leg movement, Clarkson's study investigated next how these central nervous system changes affect speed of movement and reaction time. "Other studies have shown that reaction time slows with aging, and we found that this slowing occurred predominantly in the central nervous system, not in the muscle itself. From the time the subject sees the light to the time the muscle responds, there is slowing. We are not sure exactly where this occurs but think that it probably is in the brain. Brain cells, of course, initiate movement, and because we lose an enormous number of brain cells over many years of living, there could be a change because of this loss. It could also be that the process of decision making slows as we get older. There is a decrease somewhere in central processing time, and the muscles apparently cannot compensate. So even if we do a lot of strength training and have our muscles look better, it may not help our nervous system."

balance and coordination

These changes in movement and reaction time have a strong effect on balance and coordination. Clarkson points out that most injuries older people suffer are the result of falling. "Older people fall, and fall more often, because they stumble and cannot recover like younger persons because reaction is not quick enough. Adding to the problem is decreased muscle strength and poorer balance. You need strong, reliable muscles to 'grab' you when you are about to fall. The combination of changes in central nervous system speed and loss of muscle strength is clearly there and has an impact on the older person's life. Surveys found that 24% of men and 44% of women over 65 gave a history of falls. That means over one third of this population falls, and a fall is recorded if it requires at least one day of hospitalization. There is a high incidence of hip and wrist fractures among the elderly resulting from these falls, and for many life changes drastically due to hip fractures. Staying active can have great impact on the maintenance of muscle strength, coordination, and reaction time to help avoid these kinds of accidents, one very important reason for staying fit."

Clarkson believes there needs to be stronger emphasis on maintenance of strength in aging. "It is not necessary to do weight lifting, but basic calisthenic exercises are important. Group exercise programs, in my opinion, are a wonderful solution. 'High tech' equipment is not appropriate nor does it appeal to an older population. But fitness classes for seniors can be planned to incorporate the types of activities which are important to keep up with. Safety, well-being, and overall good health should be the focus of such programs. If older people can be supported in maintaining a good level of fitness, there will be many benefits. Beyond the important factors of safety and injury-prevention, being fit will allow them to enjoy doing other active things. Instead of becoming observers, people can continue to participate in life and won't get tired doing something extra. They will have more fun, enjoy their retirement years more fully, and experience a very different quality of life."

Basically, exercise physiologists agree with what our grandparents already knew: movement is basic to life and wellness. "There is nothing very grand to say about this," Clarkson says. "It helps to scientifically understand what the problems are so that you can reasonably attack and correct them. I see older people giving up a lot of things they used to do because they no longer have the same body confidence and are afraid of getting hurt. Regular exercise continued into older age can help maintain this physical self-confidence so that life can be enjoyed more fully."

An individual's level of coordination, strength, and endurance, and the ability to react all affect daily life. Activities that maintain or enhance these capabilities are easily structured for the older individual and should be an integral part of any fitness program for this population.

bone tissue loss in aging

Bone has many functions. It provides the framework for the body, protects many of the vital organs, serves as a system of levers for movement, and helps to balance the amount of calcium and phosphorus in the body.

Osteoporosis is a big word, and a relatively new one to the layman's vocabulary. Medical concerns about osteoporosis have gained wide public awareness in the recent past. This bone disease, which causes an estimated half million to one million fractures of the wrist, hip, and spine each year, is a serious health hazard that concerns all women, young and old. Hip fractures, especially, present the most common health problem for older women, often replacing independent living with nursing home care.

Osteoporosis literally means "porous bones." Once-sturdy bones become lighter and more fragile, their interiors more like honeycombs than the solid, strong structures they once were. Bone is living tissue and is always "under construction." Calcium is removed from the bone, and new calcium is laid down; it's a continual remodeling process that takes place throughout life. From birth to early adulthood, more bone tissue is produced than is lost. A strong skeleton grows with new tissue constantly being added to the outer surfaces of the bones. But once this growth stops, a slow and steady process of bone tissue loss begins for both sexes in their early 30s.

In his recent book *Stand Tall!—The Informed Woman's Guide to Preventing Osteoporosis*, author Morris Notelovitz, MD, explains that women lose bone much more rapidly than men do. By the age of 80, a woman will have lost 47% of bone mass compared to only a 14% loss for men. Especially after menopause, women lose bone tissue twice as fast as men with the most rapid loss occurring during the first 5 to 6 years after menopause. Bone loss begins to slow again at around age 65, becoming similar to that of men. But women have already lost a great deal more than men at this time, and even though this loss slows from here on in, women's bones are now brittle and less able to withstand the physical stresses of everyday living. A simple sneeze, a misstep, lifting a heavy bag of groceries, or tripping over a rug can break one of the bones most vulnerable to osteoporosis: the wrist, spinal vertebrae, or hip.

About 200,000 hip fractures from falls are estimated to occur in 1985. Most of the patients will be women over 70, and up to 20% will die from complications. As many as half will no longer be able to live independently and will spend the rest of their lives in nursing homes. Fractures of the spinal vertebrae, many of them occurring from the simple stress of daily activity such as bending and lifting, will add to this statistic for women between the ages of 55 and 75. These spinal "compression fractures" cause the height loss many women experience in aging and the spinal curvature we know as the "dowager's hump." Both can cause greatly restricted mobility and chronic back pain.

prevention and treatment of osteoporosis

Osteoporosis is irreversible, and preventive measures begun in early adulthood and continued throughout life are the only answer to this often debilitating bone disease. Most women have a lifelong chronically inadequate intake of dietary calcium. We make sure our kids drink enough milk to build strong bones, but as adults we neglect this good advice for our own bone health. Milk and other dairy products, the major calcium sources in our diet, are often all but eliminated by calorie-conscious women, and this inadequate calcium intake is a major cause of bone demineralization. Because calcium is needed in the bloodstream for nerve transmission, muscle contraction, and blood clotting, the body will draw calcium from the "bone bank" where 98% of our calcium is stored. If not enough calcium comes in to maintain bone strength and keep blood calcium levels normal, slow and steady loss of bone tissue will continue year after year. Dr. Notelovitz's book and other current research materials provide important information to share in younger classes with women who can still take important preventive measures in the years ahead.

But what do you do when you are older and already have developed osteoporosis? No treatment can straighten a dowager's hump or help regain lost height. But bone loss can be slowed and bone mass can even increase, according to researchers. Their recommendations suggest an intake of 1,200 to 1,500 milligrams of calcium and 400 units of vitamin D daily after menopause, preferably from dietary sources. Large amounts of protein, red meat, coffee, salt, and fiber are labelled "bone robbers" by Dr. Notelovitz because they interfere with the body's ability to absorb calcium. Exercise makes a significant contribution to maintaining strong bones.

exercise and osteoporosis

Exercise is important because physical stress can actually cause bones to become stronger and denser, especially when combined with enough calcium in the diet. Calcium is deposited in proportion to the physical stress placed on bones, and researchers encourage women to participate in weight-bearing activities. Studies have shown that exercise—as little as 30 minutes three times a week—increases bone mass, even in women in their 80s. Dr. Everett Smith, who has conducted such studies at the University of Wisconsin Medical School, states that age does not seem to be a major limiting factor in the bone's response to stress. It's simple enough: All parts of the body, including bones, are dependent on movement to maintain strength and integrity.

Here, too, our programs can make a significant contribution, giving people these two structured hours of important exercise that can affect their health in so many different ways. And even though most women in our programs may already be affected by osteoporosis, they should be able to safely participate in the suggested activities. Weight-bearing activities are most important, so keeping people on their feet for a good part of the class hour is best. In addition, encourage everyone to get out for their daily walks. Explaining the important effects walking can have on keeping bones strong may give everyone the added incentive to go out with conviction. Jogging is not recommended for persons with osteoporosis because the jarring motion can traumatize already fragile bones.

posture

A friend who graduated from Smith College 25 years ago told me about a course she and all freshmen had to take at that time. It was called Basic Motor Skills and started with being photographed nude. The photos were analyzed with comments such as "You have a forward head" or "Notice your concave chest!" Those who slumped and slouched were given corrective exercises, and before a student graduated, she had to pass the posture test. Many students lived in fear of these photos falling into the hands of Amherst or Williams College men, especially before the "bad curves" were made good. At Vassar, another friend took a similar course. Women graduating from these respected institutions were expected to do so properly aligned.

Of all the body functions affected by exercise, particularly as we grow older, posture is a significant one. We cannot hold ourselves in good alignment if muscles are weak. Strong back muscles keep the spine erect and help prevent back problems and a variety of "bad curves" that make us look older than we need to. Keeping all muscles in good tone helps prevent rounded shoulders that make us look dejected and "blue," create muscle tension in upper back and neck, and cause clothes to fit poorly. An erect spine allows lungs to expand and work efficiently and the digestive system to function better. Good overall strength and mobility help prevent a hesitant, shuffling walking pattern, which makes us look old. Good posture makes us feel confident and tall: We walk with assured steps, feel safe, and present ourselves to the world around us as positive and happy people.

There are good and bad ways to walk, stand, sit, bend, and lift, and the area most likely to suffer the consequences of poor carriage and bad habits is the back. Discs between spinal vertebrae are susceptible to injury if we don't protect them, and the way we carry ourselves in the course of a lifetime can strongly affect our well-being. Bad posture places stresses on muscles, ligaments, and the spinal column, and regular exercise can do much to help prevent these discomforts and pains. Keeping back, abdominal, and hip muscles in good condition is possible at every age, and when all muscle groups are balanced and function the way they are meant to, the back is much more able to withstand stresses daily living may inflict.

Lifting, bending, and pushing can injure the back if good posture is not maintained. When lifting a large or heavy object, you should bend your knees instead of leaning forward from the waist with straight legs. Keep the back straight and the object you are lifting close to your body, and face what you are lifting squarely— never lift from a twisted position. The more you depend on your arms and legs to help with lifting, the more protected your back will be. Broaden the base of your support by having feet apart for better stability. In our class, just as we practice safely getting down to and up from the floor, we practice the body mechanics of correct lifting and bending for tasks that need to be performed.

Considering that we spend almost one-third of our lives asleep, paying attention to sleeping position is important, too. An old mattress can turn into a comfortable nest to crawl into, but for back support a firm mattress is best. Back sufferers should put a plywood board under the mattress to keep it from sagging where the body weight concentrates. Sleeping on your side with knees slightly drawn up makes for a good night's rest, whereas sleeping on your stomach exaggerates the curve of the lower back and places the neck in an awkward position. People who wake up with stiff necks may want to invest in a down pillow that conforms to head and neck, providing comfortable support. Sleeping on your back is the next best body position, especially if a pillow is placed under the knees to help straighten out the spine.

A number of my older students' posture impresses me as truly regal. They walk, stand, and sit tall and well aligned, and when I comment on their youthful carriage, it usually turns out that a nagging parent had quite an effect on their posture awareness. One 70-year-old woman vividly remembers her father's constant reminders to sit straight at the dinner table and to walk proud and tall the rest of the time. It's apparent that mothers and fathers have been posture ogres for generations. In Germany where I grew up, posture was a very important issue. Sitting at the dinner table meant sitting tall and straight. There was always the suggestion that some day we might find ourselves dining with the Queen of England and that it would be terribly embarrassing to have our heads hanging in the royal soup. Our food was simply not served unless we sat straight and displayed good manners. Although my mother knew little about the effects of poor posture on muscles, bones, and organs, she did know that slouching and slumping left a poor impression and found that reason enough to remind us over and over again. And it worked.

characteristics of good posture

What are the characteristics of good posture? Many people think of the West Point stance, the ramrod look with shoulders square and thrown back, chin tucked in so tight that the back of the neck aches. But even at West Point, where posture has been a major concern for the past 170 years, there has been a revision in that department. A person with good posture looks natural. When aligned well, the body is balanced, overall movement is efficient, muscle energy is conserved, and we don't experience fatigue. Posture basically starts in the head: Becoming aware of how we carry ourselves is the first step to making necessary corrections. Practice the mechanics of good posture occasionally with your students while walking or standing, and give these pointers:

1. Think tall and straight! Lengthen the waist and straighten the spine by pulling abdominal muscles in and lifting the chest.
2. Hold your head high, chin pointing straight ahead.
3. Shoulders are down, back, and relaxed, elongating the neck.
4. Weight is slightly forward, not back on the heels. The whole body feels relaxed and well aligned. The overall feeling is one of having a string attached to the top of the head and being pulled up toward the ceiling.

characteristics of poor posture

The most common "bad curves" are a round upper back, or a swayback. The main reason for poor posture in general is dominance of one muscle group over another. Our muscles work in opposite but cooperative pairs. When the back muscles stretch, for example, abdominal muscles contract—as in sit-ups. When the back muscles contract, the abdominal muscles stretch, as happens in standing. Unless the abdominal muscles are exercised, they begin to weaken and sag, causing an increased curve in the lower back, and the result is an unattractive swayback. A rounded upper back is often caused by many years of working at a desk or drawing board, for example. With much hunching and bending forward, shoulder girdle and upper back muscles stretch, becoming too long, and chest muscles shorten. Poor posture awareness, and not caring enough about how we carry ourselves, add to the problem—and that's where parents' reminders tend to be effective while we are young and developing good or bad habits.

Often, posture deteriorates as a result of normal aging. Bones soften and muscles are weaker and less flexible, especially if we don't resume an active life. The chin begins to jut forward, the upper back can become humped, and there is a change in how we walk and stand. We begin to shuffle, and the overall picture is no longer a youthful one. Changing eyesight adds to the problem, with a tendency to look down to make sure there are no obstacles in the way. Osteoporosis weakens bones, and fractures of the vertebrae cause women especially to become stooped from the waist up. You probably have heard older people comment that they have grown shorter, and there can be a height loss of 4 or more inches as a result of these fractures that can cause the spinal column to collapse onto itself.

On the whole, it certainly is better to develop good posture early in life and maintain it rather than suffer the physical and cosmetic discomforts in the later years when structural changes are often there to stay. Not only can round shoulders cause painful muscle tension, but shortening of the chest muscles also cramps the lungs. The "forward head" often goes along with a rounded upper back, and it looks awkward. This unnatural head position causes fatigue, neck and shoulder pain, and headaches.

improving posture

Improved posture can make a great difference in making a protruding abdomen less evident. In our class, we practice this very consciously. Place your hands on your abdomen while you are standing, and let yourself go into a comfortable slump, shoulders rounding forward. You immediately feel a handful of protruding abdomen. And now think TALL: Imagine the string attached to the top of your head, pulling you up to feel tall and erect. There is an immediate lifting of the rib cage, the neck elongates, shoulders are down and back, and the spine straightens. The waistline feels trimmer, and—voila!—the protruding abdomen disappears (more or less, depending on fatty deposits in this area). These practices are very helpful for developing greater postural awareness for daily living. If a lack of body awareness or posture concern is apparent, try to help your students develop it by appealing to their vanity. Ask them to take a good look at themselves in pro-

file at home in a full-length mirror or in store windows as they walk along. Would they pass the Smith College posture test? And what can reasonably be done at this stage in life to make a difference? Regular exercises to strengthen and stretch affected muscle groups will help greatly, and many of the exercises contained in this guide serve the purpose of improving posture. At 70, we don't expect to look as we did at 20. On the other hand, I see many teenagers with far worse posture than most of my seniors. I give constant encouragement to be aware of posture while we walk, skip, stand, or sit. It can become a new, better habit and help us to move through the day with more ease, less postural strain, and a much more youthful look.

Our vocabulary contains phrases that clearly point out signals we send to the world around us in the way we carry ourselves. "Keep your chin up," "hold your head high," "being in a slump," or "feeling down" are very descriptive of mental attitudes expressed through posture. But letting the body react to our mental states can also be turned around: We can affect the way we feel about ourselves by literally "pulling ourselves together." Walking proud and erect and looking our best gives us a physical and mental lift and makes us feel secure and self-confident. No matter what the present posture picture is, it can be improved through awareness, regular exercise to strengthen and stretch important muscle groups, and the development of better habits throughout every day. Figure faults are less noticeable if proud posture is what impresses those around us, no matter how old we are.

I encourage my students to spend a few minutes every day with some very simple posture exercises:

1. Stand erect and hold hands behind the back. Tighten buttock and abdominal muscles, then straighten the arms and pull them away from the back. This creates a strong stretch across chest and shoulders and is a good reminder especially for those with a tendency to slump into a round-shouldered position.
2. Place a broomstick behind shoulder blades and spend a few minutes daily walking tall and erect, chest open and chin up.
3. After taking a bath, hold the bath towel overhead, arms straight and long, towel tightly stretched. Tighten buttock and abdominal muscles, and pull arms back to stretch rib cage, waist, and shoulders.
4. To strengthen and shorten the shoulder girdle, place hands against a wall at shoulder level, standing about 3 ft away. Tighten buttock and abdominal muscles and bend elbows to bring the chin to the wall, keeping body tight and in a straight line. Push away to straighten arms again, and repeat 10 times.

5. To stretch out low back muscles next, lie on your back. Draw one knee close to your chest, lifting head and shoulders, and hold for a few seconds. Relax, and repeat with other leg. Repeat this stretching exercise several times.

6. For an overall stretch, stay on your back and hold hands above your head. Straighten arms, feeling rib cage and waistline lengthen, and push away with heels to stretch hips and legs.

It takes so little time to help ourselves move through the day with more ease and grace, feeling light on our feet and confident in our stride. Encourage your students to spend these few minutes daily to look and feel their best.

There is overall agreement among professionals involved in researching the various aspects of aging that the maintenance of a generally healthy, active lifestyle is essential if we want to keep quality in our lives as we grow older. Research in the field of exercise physiology will continue to further our knowledge and motivate us more strongly to stay physically active so that we can enjoy the years ahead feeling well and energetic, remain productive, and minimize some of the degeneration that makes us feel and look older than we need to.

11
medical concerns in aging

Aging is an ongoing progression of biological changes, affecting all types of cells and tissues. Decline in ability and physical signs of aging appear as we grow older, but these changes vary greatly from one person to another. Aging is a lifelong process and takes place at different rates for different individuals. These individual variations are there at every age but become more pronounced in the older years. Genetics, medical history, lifelong exercise and food habits, environmental stress, social, cultural, and psychological experiences all play a role in the aging process; each life history is unique to the individual. As a result, there is more diversity among older people than any other age group, and blanket statements about function, ability, and health in the older years should not be made.

There are, however, certain normal and common changes in health status as we age. As one medical friend put it, "The body slowly starts to wear out from many years of use. The longer you live, the more likely you are to experience some of these degenerative changes. Don't expect to get older without aches, pains, and certain limitations. But don't let it stop you from continuing to enjoy an active, high-quality life. It's not activity that gets people into trouble, but giving in and giving up does!"

One factor which is very much in our favor as we conduct fitness programs for seniors is that there is a process of self-selection. Those who join our programs have made this decision because they feel well and capable enough to participate. Persons with real handicaps or seriously impaired health will not be likely to join such activities. Those who do come have been encouraged to do so by their personal physicians or have the desire to take this very positive step because they understand that exercise is important for maintaining long-term wellness and good health. Their mental outlook is positive, and their health status makes such decision making realistic. It should be emphasized again that the exercise materials contained in this manual are intended for the large segment of the older population that is in possession of overall good health rather than those in need of other approaches, such as physical therapy or individualized exercise prescription, due to more serious physical limitations or health problems.

Many of those we will see in our classes have never ceased to pursue an active, healthy lifestyle. They have taken responsibility for their continued wellness through the middle years, and the transition into older age has been smooth and normal. They are realistic about normal wear and tear, informed and knowledgeable about whatever medical condition may exist, and not foolhardy in their participation. They make good decisions based on medical advice and take responsibility for staying well, independent, and fully functional as long as possible. We should strongly support and encourage these people in our programs. In addition, we can help those who are taking the first steps away from a sedentary existence. Each participant has the opportunity to explore his or her individual physical potential safely and positively as long as we respect this individuality within the framework of our programs and are knowledgeable about the effects of exercise on various common conditions.

"I cannot think of any condition which would not benefit from appropriate movement," one medical friend commented. Whether it be arthritis, high blood pressure, respiratory ailments, or other problems that have developed, the human body was made to move and all systems depend on movement to function as well as possible. If intensity is appropriately adjusted and individual limitations taken into account, a person in his or her 60s or 70s should be able to do what was possible in the younger years. We have to get away from the dominant impression that growing older, in itself, inflicts decline, frailty, ill health, and severe physical limitations. The majority of older persons do not fall into this category and are perfectly capable of participating in sensible activity. We cannot hope to address everyone's needs in our programs, but we can work with the many who possess the desire and capacity to make the most of the years ahead. It is challenging and satisfying to mobilize the unused or underused potential older adults possess and to help influence attitudes, physical self-confidence, vitality, and lifestyles. The capacity each person has to improve his or her well-being can be of greater significance than what medical care may provide, especially if we believe in prevention as being preferable to cure. Good medical care, of course, is of vital importance but cannot be a substitute for continued good self-care and a generally healthy, active life-

style. It's how we live on a daily basis that gives us the energy, vitality, and wellness we desire for the later years, and medicine cannot offer a better substitute.

maintaining a positive attitude toward wellness

As I look through books discussing health in midlife and beyond, it becomes clear that it would be easy to get quite discouraged. There are failing eyesight and hearing, hardening of the arteries, arthritis, back problems, bunions, depression, and loss of memory, to name just a few. The human body is a vast reservoir of potential problems, and if we become preoccupied with the possibility of becoming victims of these conditions, it's easy to see old age as not worth living for. Bookshelves even offer formidable encyclopaedias of symptoms for self-diagnosis, and by surrounding ourselves with such materials, we can easily become submerged in waves of fear, finding something new and different wrong as each day passes. It's time for materials that take a more encouraging look at health in the older years, showing us the control we have over many aspects of our health and the aging process. We need to be informed and encouraged, not discouraged, so we can expect to feel well and keep losses and changes to a reasonable minimum.

You will encounter this positive attitude among the participants with whom you work. Their ability to minimize problems that have developed, rather than dwell on them, is often remarkable. They don't give in or give up but instead fight to maintain a solid grip on wellness. They don't have unreasonable expectations and accept the changes that are part and parcel of living long. They seek good medical care, follow medical advice, and live sensibly. They don't look for new symptoms but expect to avoid them if at all possible, maintain a positive mental outlook, and focus on the good things in their lives.

exercise-oriented physicians

Dr. Mark Peterman is an internist here in Amherst, and many participants in my program are under his care. He is a committed and enthusiastic exerciser and knows from personal experience how much regular activity can affect the quality of a person's life. His personal beliefs carry over into his practice where he educates his patients in lifestyle changes and self-responsibility, and strongly encourages making time for sensible, regular exercise at every age. An exercise-oriented physician can have great influence on patients who lead sedentary lives. There is personal experience and conviction behind his advice to exercise, and it has the power to impress. Dr. Peterman made clear that having a good program in the community to direct patients to is very helpful and much more valuable than the standard advice to get some exercise, which usually results in patients' doing nothing. A structured program is what most people need to make a commitment to regular activity, and if the program is sensible and appropriate, physicians are glad to urge their older patients to participate.

Physicians in internal medicine tend to take care of a middle-aged and older population. "After the age of about 50, some conditions are accelerated," Dr. Peterman explained. "In the 50s, 60s, and 70s we see much heart disease and other degenerative conditions. The body is showing signs of wearing out. In addition to heart disease, the vascular system shows degeneration, and anything that moves shows wear and tear." The years between 20 and 40 tend to be relatively healthy ones with few serious problems. But at around age 40, his patients start to get overweight, have elevated blood pressure, and show early signs of other degenerative diseases. "At that point I start some serious lifestyle counseling," he said. "With middle-aged patients, I practice preventive medicine. I make sure they don't have blood disorders or chronic diseases. Most of them are healthy at this point, and I spend a lot of time encouraging them to exercise, watch their diets, and take care of their bodies. I hand responsibility to them. Their health will be as good as their daily habits. People in their 70s are not likely to reverse chronic conditions which have developed since midlife. Midlife is the time to take action and responsibility, rather than depending on medical treatments for problems in the older years."

But even though chronic conditions cannot be reversed at age 70, there can be a great difference in the quality of life. "The dye has been cast by the way we have lived. But even though degeneration is taking place, the quality of life can be high in spite of these conditions. When I look at patients who come into my office smiling and positive, they are the people who are still active, walking, or working physically, not those who sit in front of their television sets all day long. It seems to me that the happy people are active people, that their mental well-being is strongly affected by their level of physical involvement. They are consciously trying to do something about preserving their physical abilities and independence and take responsibility for their wellness."

individual exercise advice

According to Dr. Peterman, people who don't like to exercise don't bring up the subject. The patients who want to discuss exercise tend to be middle-aged, concerned about their present lifestyle, and afraid that they might have a heart attack if they begin an exercise program. "But not many of my older patients bring up the subject of exercise. I have to do it," he pointed out. "For people in their 60s and 70s, it's very helpful if the physician urges them into a more active lifestyle and makes clear how much they have to gain from staying active and fit, both physically and psychologically. I believe that a great part of older people's happiness comes from exercising and feeling well as a result. This belief makes me urge and encourage my older patients into regular, sensible exercise, and I make a point of discussing it during office visits."

When asked how much he feels people in general are influenced by medical advice to exercise, Dr. Peterman's matter-of-fact reply was, "A lot less than we physicians like to believe, especially if people are on their own with an exercise program. Even those who catch the fever and will keep it up for a number of months tend to be back to sedentary living when I see them a year later. They may have gotten off track because something major has happened in their lives or because it simply isn't a priority. It's mostly a matter of people's psyche, and they may see problems in their lives as so overwhelming that exercise seems like one more major effort to have to make. They want to retreat into a cocoon—read, watch TV, go to bed, and tune out. If people would give themselves a chance and discover the outlet and great energy you get from regular exercise, their motivation to continue would be stronger. But it's tough to tell a nonexerciser how good exercise can feel. It has to be a positive personal experience, and an organized class with good leadership can provide an important start for many who are not self-motivated."

When it comes to individual exercise advice, Dr. Peterman finds it most important to look at what the person would enjoy doing. "Basically, I encourage all patients to keep moving, stay as active as possible in their daily lives, and exercise in whatever way they most enjoy it. If they don't enjoy what they are doing, they won't set aside the time for it." Rhythmic exercise, walking, swimming, or biking are the staple activities available to an older age group. The socialization and interaction offered in an organized fitness class can make exercise time more enjoyable for many than can the more solitary activities. "An indoor program is a great help once bad weather sets in. It gets dark early, sidewalks and roads are icy, and walking is not safe for an older person. For those who rely on walking for exercise, it may mean that activity is suddenly taken away unless they can join an indoor program where there is light, heat, and a roof over everyone's head. And as is true for younger people, too, it helps a great deal to have group support when it comes to exercise. It encourages greater commitment and long-term adherence."

medical clearance to exercise

As advising physician for a local health club, Dr. Peterman has signed many medical release forms over the years. "But I know that the people who run this facility are very knowledgeable and oriented to working with individuals. I can be sure that my middle-aged patients who join will be carefully monitored during and after exercise because professionals are working with them. It's important to distinguish between exercise programs for a middle-aged population and activities appropriate for seniors. I would certainly not release an older patient to a program of weight lifting, for example, nor do I find a jogging program appropriate for older, sedentary patients. But I would have to say that I am more concerned about careful screening and monitoring of middle-aged persons with heart disease risk factors as they begin an exercise program than I am about a relatively healthy older person who is not likely to engage in overly stressful activity."

For the 40-year-old, he explained, it is important to be educated about the guidelines established for safe cardiovascular exercise, especially if there are risk factors to be concerned about. He teaches patients to take their pulse and gives basic advice to follow so that true aerobic conditioning can take place. "Much has been published recently about risk of sudden death during exercise, especially after Jim Fixx died while running. This risk is anywhere from 5 to 20 times higher when you are exercising strenuously, and the lower percentage applies even to conditioned athletes. But that certainly doesn't mean people should not exercise! It's important to look at the level and regularity of exertion. The statistics of a 20-time increased risk of sudden death applies to the person who has done absolutely nothing and then goes out and tries to run 5 miles or starts a strenuous weight-lifting program. From nothing to too much—that's where risk enters into the picture. But if a person is already walking regularly and decides to start a sensible walk/jog program, the chances of suffering detrimental results are very minimal." Dr. Peterman's concern about the national frenzy in the exercise movement again applies to a middle-aged rather than an older patient population because they are more influenced by it and may suffer serious health consequences by being pushed into more than they can handle. "It's impossible to make a blanket statement about the issue of medical release forms. I certainly would not sign such a form for a program I am not fully informed about. Signing a release basically expresses my total agreement with the patient's participation, and such agreement can only exist if I know the program to be safe and good. There is too much fad exercising out there, and I want patients to stay away from the excess which is presently so in vogue. I would much rather see them engage in reasonable exercise, such as brisk walking or light jogging, where there is no need for a release form."

Medical release forms typically involve a thorough physical examination and perhaps exercise stress testing. The older patient who wants to join a fitness class or begin a sensible program of individual activity should not be discouraged from these good intentions by insisting on either, Dr. Peterman feels. It would be unusual for a 70-year-old person to engage in a level of activity that could be detrimental. "At this older age, I don't worry so much about heart rate monitoring or following specific guidelines. I tell my patients to just get out and get their blood moving and work up a bit of perspiration. The amount of time these people spend with exercise is more important than the intensity. If they want to stimulate their cardiovascular system, they should get out and move for at least one-half hour three to four times a week. It's important that they spend enough time at a stretch to get a moderate workout instead of just taking a leisurely walk around the block for a few minutes. The amount of time they devote to exercise is more important to me from a medical standpoint than their exercise pulse rate. At 70, we no longer look at exercise as long-term aerobic conditioning; we just want to keep people moving and feeling well. There's no need to get neurotic about pulse-taking, or to get afraid of the physiology of what happens during exercise and stop as a result. More than anything else, I want my older patients to enjoy exercise and keep it up, whatever form that may take. I stress *moderation and regularity*. People need to first look at what they are used to doing, and add on to that in reasonable increments. Excessive exercise is what can hurt and injure instead of doing good. But as long as things are kept at a sensible level—and most older people will do just that—we should be supportive and not get hung up on expensive physicals, stress testing, release forms, and pulse rate monitoring which may discourage participation at an older age. There is, of course, a need to be very familiar with the patient's profile and health history so that the medical advice for exercise is well-founded. Over the years, I have only kept one patient from exercising because his blood pressure was dangerously high and needed to be brought under control first. But even this one case was only a temporary situation, and he returned to activity as soon as his blood pressure was down. The typical degenerative conditions we see in our older patients simply do not prevent reasonable exercise participation. From a physician's standpoint, I can only be supportive of getting people out of their rocking chairs so that they feel better all around and slow down the process of aging and degeneration."

arthritis

Arthritis is one of the oldest diseases known. Neanderthal paintings dating back more than 40,000 years show our arthritic ancestors with stooped postures and walking with bent knees. Arthritis occurs in all races at all ages, and it also occurs in animals. An estimated 40 million Americans suffer from arthritis, and almost everyone joining our programs will be affected to some degree. Arthritis is not just one disease but includes many different conditions that share common characteristics. Osteoarthritis and rheumatoid arthritis are the two types we need to understand so we can educate participants in our classes about the value and importance of continued exercise.

Simply put, arthritis means that problems have developed in one or more joints in the body. Joints are complex structures consisting of six parts, all of which can be attacked by arthritis:

- *Cartilage* covers the end of each of the two bones that meet in the joint, cushioning and protecting them and providing movement without friction.
- *Bursae* are small sacs near joints. They contain fluid that lubricates the movement of muscle across muscle or muscle across bone.
- *Synovial sacs* surround and protect joints and secrete synovial fluid, which lubricates joints.
- *Muscles* are elastic tissue and make all movement at the joints possible, shortening or lengthening to move bones.
- *Tendons* are fibrous cords attaching muscles to bones.
- *Ligaments* are fibrous, too, but much shorter than tendons, and attach bone to bone.

When someone has arthritis, something is wrong with one or more of these parts. The resulting discomforts can put a real damper on a person's desire to exercise in spite of knowing that movement is essential therapy for arthritis.

osteoarthritis

Osteoarthritis is the most common variety of arthritis, the kind that catches up with all of us sooner or later, a universal condition that worsens with age. It is not very responsive to medical treatment, and there is no known cure. Fortunately, very few people experience severe symptoms. The tissue involved is the cartilage, tough as gristle and very durable. Cartilage does not have a blood supply, and the oxygen and nutrients it needs are supplied by the surrounding joint fluid. Cartilage is elastic and can absorb fluid. In activity, pressure of joint movement squeezes fluids and waste products out of the cartilage, and when the pressure is relieved, fluid containing nourishment and oxygen is returned. Cartilage health, therefore, depends on regular use of joints. But over many years of use, cartilage begins to fray, wear thin, or even wear away completely. Most of us will experience symptoms of this wear-and-tear condition starting in midlife. The changes occur mostly in weight-bearing joints and don't really place major limitations on activity, especially if intensity and pace are appropriately adjusted. My 68-year-old tennis partner recently decided to be more sensible and substitute some doubles matches for the hard, fast singles he loves and to stay away from hard-surface courts. His arthritic knees were beginning to bother him too much, making clear that some adjustments in exercise intensity were called for. "I want these knees to last until I'm 90," he insists, "and I love tennis too much to give it up before then!" Instead of giving in to the discomforts of arthritis and giving up his sport, he is now staying active without abusing his knees.

A joint injury can cause arthritic changes to begin even at a young age. Inactivity affects cartilage by leaving it poorly nourished. Unstable joints due to weak ligaments, tendons, and muscles may cause cartilage to wear unevenly. Being overweight and having poor posture habits may take their toll. Excessive physical stress can also cause damage to weight-bearing joints. Beyond these factors, it's simply living for many years and bearing the body's weight that causes joint degeneration.

The main symptoms of osteoarthritis are creaky, stiff joints. The mildest and earliest form of this joint problem occurs in the last joints of the fingers. As a sort of defense against arthritis, the body often builds up little deposits of bone around these joints, and these small swellings at the side of the joints are characteristic of osteoarthritis and are called Heberden's nodes. This arthritis is often hereditary and primarily affects middle-aged women whose mothers or grandmothers may have had it. It tends to subside on its own after a period of swelling and tenderness, leaving behind knobby joints and stiffness but little pain.

Primary osteoarthritis occurs with progressing age. It can start as early as 40 but mostly affects people after 60. Knees and hip joints work strenuously year after year and are the second most common joints affected. As cartilage wears down, joint space is reduced and the joint is less efficient in function. At first things feel uncomfortable and stiff, and then there is pain. The knees often produce grating sounds as rough cartilage grinds together. Continued movement lubricates this injured joint and keeps it functional. For many older folks, arthritis in the knees may produce enough pain to limit range of movement. Weakening of surrounding muscles and other connective tissue can leave the knee joint unstable and cause the feeling that the knee will buckle. Just as it does in affected finger joints, the body may lay down bony deposits in the knee, which can result in swelling, stiffness, discomfort, and decreased mobility. Maintaining normal weight is one sensible preventive measure, reducing the amount of stress on weight-bearing joints and on the lower back.

Osteoarthritis of the hip tends to be most disabling because the pain and stiffness can interfere greatly with everyday living. All weight-bearing activities, getting into and out of chairs, climbing stairs, or getting into the tub, can become difficult tasks. But there is positive intervention for those who become seriously limited by the progression of this condition. When the joint becomes too diseased, an orthopaedic surgeon will consider replacing the hip with an artificial one. Surgery is followed by a period of physical therapy to strengthen muscles, ligaments, and tendons, and the person returns to normal activity, happy to be pain-free and with better range of motion than the diseased joint allowed. Several of my students have a new hip, and their level of participation is impressive. They have physical confidence because the joint replacement is stable and dependable, and its construction allows normal range of movement. Two women in our class have undergone surgery to replace a diseased knee joint, and both agree that they are somewhat anxious to have their surgeons agree to replacing the other knee, also. Hip or knee replacement does not seem to limit these people's participation in our program, other than their staying away from jumping or similar activities that place too much stress on weight-bearing joints. But here again, individuals know their limits, and they simply avoid the activities that are not comfortable or safe.

rheumatoid arthritis

Rheumatoid arthritis is quite different from osteoarthritis. It can appear early in life and is more common in women than men. There is active inflammation of the lining of the joints and other connective tissues. It is caused by an inflammatory reaction in the joints and can start slowly or appear very suddenly. The middle joints of the fingers tend to be affected first, causing tenderness and swelling. As the condition progresses, wrists, ankles, knees, elbows, and shoulders may become involved. Symptoms include swelling, stiffness,

pain, and limited range of motion. Movement may aggravate the pain in the early stages, and rest brings relief. As the disease progresses, stiffness and pain are the major complaints, and they are worst after periods of rest, especially in the mornings, and improve with movement. Medical treatment includes the use of anti-inflammatory agents and medications to bring pain relief. Physical therapy and exercise approaches have to include a careful balance of activity and rest to keep joints mobile and surrounding tissues strong and elastic without undue stress. The active phase of rheumatoid arthritis will subside over a period of weeks or months, and physical therapy or appropriate exercise are important treatments in retaining function and mobility. Those not severely affected by this condition participate with medical guidance and know by being in touch with their condition how much exercise is appropriate.

Sensible exercise is of crucial importance to prevent the loss of function that may accompany arthritis. The "use it or lose it" principle has great meaning. If muscles and joints are not used consistently, there will be loss of strength, mobility, and function. The only time joints should be rested is during inflammatory stages, but even then gentle range of motion exercises are strongly advised.

Unfortunately, many people with arthritis think that exercise may be harmful because it often is accompanied by pain. It's easy to become discouraged, and in our class settings we can offer the necessary support to help those with problems. The numerous benefits of exercise touch many aspects of a person's life, both physically and psychologically. Being in charge of maintaining function and independence and knowing that movement nourishes the diseased joints can be highly motivating in spite of the discomforts often associated with exercise. It's important to feel a sense of control and accomplishment rather than passively accepting a condition that can be slowed and improved by taking responsibility and staying active.

Dr. Peterman feels that those with arthritic conditions should remain as active as is reasonably possible. "What needs to be understood is that without regular movement, contractures of tissues surrounding the joints can occur. Muscles and tendons atrophy, bones start to stick together, and then there is little that can be done. Even though we cannot improve the diseased condition of the joint through exercise, it is crucial to retain the fullest possible range of motion. The underlying disease will continue, but exercise will help greatly in reducing complications. I see little reason for not remaining as active as possible and strongly encourage this. Obviously, the person with diseased knees or hips should not begin a jogging program or engage in stressful activities such as jumping or weight lifting. But they will do fine with swimming, walking, using an exercise bike, or participating in rhythmic range of motion activities. Depending on the degree of discomfort, swimming is always a positive solution because it is non-weight bearing and easier on the joints. If exercise participation causes lasting discomfort, it is important to make adjustments in exercise intensity. On the whole, I recommend that people exercise within their personal limits and stretch that limit just a little more each time. My advice again is regularity and moderation, and people will find that with time they can do more than they expected. You simply have to be sensible and use good judgment, look at what you are used to doing, and slowly add on to this present level of physical activity. Following the 'train, don't strain' advice is important, and exercise will then be experienced as helpful and enjoyable."

high blood pressure (hypertension)

About 75% of those affected by high blood pressure are over 40, even though it can also seriously affect younger people. Because it is very likely that some of your students will have elevated blood pressure, there is a need to be informed about this condition to help make exercise a safe and beneficial experience.

Simply put, high blood pressure means that the pressure of blood within the blood vessels is higher than it should be. When blood pressure readings are taken, the higher figure expresses the systolic pressure, the pressure in the arteries at the height of each contraction of the heart muscle as it pumps blood. The lower figure is the diastolic pressure, which is measured when the heart relaxes to fill with blood and rests between beats. This diastolic pressure is the measure of constant minimal pressure in the arteries. In general, the systolic reading should be below 140 millimeters of mercury and the diastolic pressure below 90. The higher the reading, the greater are the possibilities that hypertension may in time damage vital organs.

factors influencing blood pressure

A number of factors may raise blood pressure by causing blood vessels to harden or narrow, making passage of blood more difficult. "Let's look at the extreme of a 10-year-old," Dr. Peterman explained. "When we look at that young person's blood vessels during contractions of the heart, we see that the vessels actually pulsate and get bigger as if to absorb some of this pumping force. Healthy arteries are distensible organs; they are flexible and allow blood to pass through with ease. What we see in older patients is that vessels have hardened and are more like rigid pipes; they no

longer expand as they should during peak pressure. It is common to see elevated systolic pressure with a normal diastolic reading, and that is called systolic hypertension of the elderly."

When blood pressure is elevated, the body is faced with a real problem. The amount of blood and fluids within the vessels is too great relative to the openings of these vessels. Abnormal pressure against the arterial walls is generated as the heart tries to force blood through these rigid openings, and this constant stress can do serious damage. "It causes wear and tear on end organs," explained Dr. Peterman, "especially the brain, heart, and kidneys. The kidneys react to high pressure over a long period of time by undergoing scarring changes, and this is a significant cause of kidney disease in the elderly. In the brain, this high pressure can cause accelerated atherosclerosis and ultimate clotting in an artery. It can increase the risk of cerebral hemorrhage, and of the different types of strokes, this is the worst kind to have because it is often progressive and can be fatal. The heart itself gets worn out because it has to constantly work against this high pressure. And in a general sense, there is a direct relationship throughout the entire body between high blood pressure and acceleration of atherosclerosis. Anybody who is prone to atherosclerosis will experience it more severely if high blood pressure is present."

There are a number of factors which contribute to the development of hypertension. "Smoking is a serious factor," Dr. Peterman pointed out. "Smoking restricts blood vessels and increases peripheral resistance by releasing adrenaline, which makes vessels clamp down. As soon as you smoke a cigarette, you can see the rise in blood pressure. Coffee, because it is a stimulant to the cardiovascular system, is another factor, and so is stress. Then there is salt intake, causing fluid retention and increasing fluid volume in the arteries. Even if blood vessels are of a normal size, this fluid increase creates problems. The best example would be the build-up of pressure in a garden hose if you try to get too much water through. We Americans have a very high salt intake. Many people are not affected by this. Their kidneys reject the overload of salt, and it is lost through urination. But other kidneys hang on to salt, and then it becomes important to shake the salt habit. We also need to add obesity to the list, and reducing weight will reduce blood pressure. In fact, changes in any area I have mentioned can help lower blood pressure. The only problem is getting people to the point of recognizing how much responsibility and control they have over making changes in their present lifestyle, and therefore in their health."

treatments for hypertension

One serious problem with high blood pressure is that the majority of patients do not show symptoms. It is usually recognized only by blood pressure readings, and these readings become part and parcel of physical checkups, especially in midlife and beyond. Once it has been established that elevated pressure is present, patients are urged to have their blood pressure taken at regular intervals. Changes in lifestyle (smoking, salt, weight, etc.) are preferred treatment and alone may be successful in mild hypertension, and exercise, too, becomes an important part of this treatment. In more difficult cases, medication is prescribed to bring blood pressure down.

"Exercise, in my opinion, is always an important factor in conditions which can be improved by general lifestyle changes," Dr. Peterman explained, "and high blood pressure is no exception. Often people will stop smoking, eat more balanced diets, and lose weight once they get in touch with themselves physically. And exercise is invaluable in reducing stress. I can't say enough about the positive effects of regular, moderate exercise." He points out that it is important to understand that almost everyone experiences a rise in blood pressure during exercise. "It gets the system revved up and activates the pressure necessary to bring oxygen and nutrients to working muscles. It's a normal function of the body. What we need to be aware of is that there is a line at which this increase is beneficial to the system and another line at which it has the potential for causing serious problems. Let's take the example of a 70-year-old with high blood pressure who may have some frail vessels in the brain. If this person were to exercise or physically work too strenuously, blood pressure could become dangerously high and possibly burst one of these frail vessels. This is why something like weight lifting should never be undertaken. The stress of such exertion can make blood pressure skyrocket and invite disaster." Even in moderate activity, a person with serious hypertension can get into trouble, Dr. Peterman pointed out. A medical clearance is a must before engaging in exercise; very elevated blood pressure must be brought under control first. "I start to get nervous when a patient's resting systolic reading is above 165. Certainly anyone with a resting systolic pressure of around 190 should not engage in vigorous activity. The most important thing is to bring blood pressure down first. With medication, this may come about within days to weeks. But if it's mild hypertension, I certainly encourage participation in sensible, moderate exercise. It is part of the treatment and will help the person in the long run. Exercise, in addition to salt restriction, stress reduction, weight loss, and stopping

smoking, can in most cases control mild hypertension, and this treatment is certainly preferable to medication."

Dr. Peterman stresses the importance of taking responsibility for having blood pressure checked regularly once it has been shown to be elevated. Most communities offer blood pressure clinics, and at our Amherst Senior Center a nurse is available every week to take these readings. "For me as a physician, it is very helpful to have patients come in with five or six readings which have been taken during the 3-month interval, which is usual between my seeing patients with high blood pressure. I believe that persons with high blood pressure are responsible for staying in close touch with their condition and seeing their physician regularly. Consequently, they can safely participate in moderate exercise programs."

Occasionally, a person will be referred to my program who has recovered from a stroke. If the physician has given clearance for exercise participation, the person can safely join in most of our activities. There will be limitations, and these differ from one person to the next. "It is important to watch these participants closely," Dr. Peterman advised. "They should not push themselves too much, and they need to keep track of their blood pressure. Allow these people to do what they feel comfortable and safe with, to exercise within their limitations without feeling any pressure to do more than that. Poststroke patients should definitely be advised by the attending physician when it comes to exercise, but a safe group setting can be important to follow up on physical therapy treatments which have come to an end." The San Francisco Heart Association has recently developed a model program of exercise for poststroke patients, and if a similar program is offered in your area, you may want to be informed about its existence.

coronary artery disease

Coronary arteries are special supply lines that furnish blood with its oxygen and nutrients to the heart muscle. There are two sets of coronary arteries: One primarily feeds the left side of the heart, the other chiefly the right side and the back of the left side. These arteries keep the heart muscle alive and functioning, and any significant interruption in their service is a direct threat to life.

Coronary arteries are prone to narrowing and obstruction. A common disease of the coronary arteries is *atherosclerosis*, a process of plaque formation that narrows arteries. This plaque development has been found to start at a young adult age, demonstrated by autopsies of young Korean war veterans that showed the beginning of degeneration of major vessels. "It is a process of our culture and of aging," Dr. Peterman explained. "It's a lifelong process and can develop more rapidly in some people than others. By the time they are in their 40s or 50s, there can be critical narrowing of one or more coronary vessels because of this plaque buildup. When we look at such a diseased artery, it's like looking at an old lead pipe in our homes. It can be completely laden with debris, seriously restricting the blood flow to that portion of the heart muscle. The smooth inner lining of the artery becomes roughened and irregular as cholesterol is deposited in the walls and as scar tissue is formed. Clots may form on the plaques, and the result is that the artery is less flexible and its opening narrower in areas of plaque formation. A normal, healthy artery opening is slightly larger than the size of a pencil lead, but a diseased artery opening may have been reduced to the size of a pin or be completely occluded. When we do catherization of an artery, we often see just a pinhole opening for blood to go through. Obviously that blood vessel is not supplying much blood to the heart muscle. This artery can become completely blocked, chiefly when a clot forms on a plaque, plugging the opening and completely depriving a section of the heart muscle of blood and resulting in a heart attack."

angina pectoris

Angina pectoris is a common symptom indicating the presence of such obstruction in the coronary arteries and literally means "constricting pain in the chest." A diseased and obstructed artery may supply enough blood to the heart muscle at rest or during inactivity, but if the heart's work is increased through exercise, emotions, or stress, the need for blood is also increased. And if obstructed arteries cannot meet this demand for greater blood flow, the heart signals its distress in the form of angina pain. Angina is usually experienced for one to several minutes as a tightness in the middle of the chest or across the whole front of the chest and may radiate to the neck and lower jaw, the shoulders, and one or both arms. If angina pain is brought on by exertion, it is called predictable angina. It is a direct signal that the level of exertion is too great and that the heart is not receiving enough oxygen to sustain this effort.

Persons with diagnosed coronary artery disease can rely on these signals during activity, Dr. Peterman explained. "I encourage patients with predictable angina to exercise within reason. If they experience angina pain, it is a clear message that they have to adjust the level and pace of exercise. Many people have chronic predictable angina and yet lead entirely normal lives, working every day and pursuing activities

they enjoy. The majority of men over 40, and many women then and in later life, have some degree of atherosclerosis. Nature does its best to overcome the difficulty by opening new arterial branches (collateral circulation) to improve the flow of blood to the heart. Exercise participation can be instrumental in the development of this collateral circulation. Improving overall fitness through regular moderate exercise will improve circulation to the rest of the body. People who stay active will find that they can tolerate more exercise in time and experience angina less often. That's the beautiful thing about conditioning. The heart still has the same limitations because the diseased state of the arteries cannot be changed. But the rest of the body improves its ability to do more within these limitations, and there is every reason to stay active rather than being overcome by fear and leading the life of an invalid."

"In the treatment of angina in general, the most important thing is to eliminate risk factors. By stopping smoking, controlling blood pressure, reducing weight, exercising regularly, and leading a reasonably active life, a person can often improve or even eliminate painful symptoms. But it takes the patient's willingness to take responsibility and to believe in the power of these lifestyle changes, something we often have a very hard time convincing patients of."

Dr. Peterman is far more concerned about patients with unpredictable angina, those who experience angina pains even at rest. He feels that these persons should probably not exercise. "Their circulation is unstable. They may either need more medication or other aggressive treatment, but I don't think they should come to exercise programs. I wish that most people with angina would have predictable exertional angina, but unfortunately that is not always the case, and we have to be conservative and concerned about those who experience angina unpredictably."

medication for coronary heart disease

A variety of medications are used in the treatment of coronary problems, and the use of *beta blockers* is common and needs to be understood in terms of exercise participation. Beta blockers lower cardiac output and cause the heart to beat less forcefully. Heart rate is considerably lowered by beta blockers, preventing heart rate from reaching greatly accelerated levels, and people taking this medication need to be aware that their heart rate during exercise will reach only a certain upper limit. Even though guidelines established for cardiovascular conditioning suggest exercise at a certain heart rate, these recommendations cannot be the same for such persons. Dr. Peterman pointed out that even during treadmill stress testing to the point of exhaustion, the heart rate of a person treated with beta blockers cannot exceed a certain limit, and that this is the direct result of necessary medication and needs to be understood and fully respected.

Of all the fears we instructors may carry around, the greatest probably is that a person might have a heart attack while participating in our programs. "There is little evidence that I am aware of to indicate that people have heart attacks because they exercise," said Dr. Peterman. "People have heart attacks under many different circumstances. I realize that much publicity is created when someone has a heart attack on the ski slopes or while jogging, but it is important to understand that it was not primarily the exercise which brought on the problem. Heart attacks are usually caused by a blood clot lodging in an already narrowed vessel, and this can happen during sleep or at any other time. People with heart problems usually will tend to exercise to the point of angina and then stop, rather than exercising to the point of heart attack. And if exercise is of a sensible nature, the fear of it bringing on a heart attack is not reasonable. It should not serve as an excuse for sedentary living, which is certainly not health-promoting for the person with cardiovascular disease."

lifestyle and heart disease

In addition to treating patients with appropriate medications, physicians make every effort to encourage improvements in lifestyle. According to Dr. Peterman, "The major risk factors in coronary artery disease are smoking, blood pressure, and cholesterol intake, and these we can do something about. It's amazing that God gave us three risk factors in this major disease we can have control over. You can't change family history, nor whether you are male or female, but a lot of other things can be controlled. If you are overweight, you can make a change there. You can change a sedentary lifestyle and try to control high stress levels. These are the risk factors of our culture. And there is no age at which I would say that stopping smoking, especially, would not improve a person's longevity! If we look at cancer, once a person has smoked a certain amount they have made themselves vulnerable to a certain risk level of developing lung cancer. But when it comes to cardiovascular disease, risk factors are reduced the moment you stop smoking, and that is why organizations like the American Heart Association are making every effort to educate the general public. I can't say enough about how much effect smoking cessation has on reducing the risk of heart attacks and the fact that exercise participation can help greatly with this important change. What all this boils down to over and over again is that we as individuals have to take much more responsibility for maintaining our good health by the way we live on a daily basis."

respiratory conditions

With age the heart, lungs, and circulatory system gradually begin to lose some of their efficiency. Lungs become less elastic, their tiny air sacs (alveoli) thicken, and there is a slow decline in the amount of air that can be taken in and expelled. Lungs and heart are responsible for delivering oxygen and nutrients to every cell of the body and for carrying away waste products. Lungs extract oxygen from the air we breathe in and exchange it for carbon dioxide. Oxygen is the fuel muscles need for work and exercise, and our maximum breathing capacity is one of the most critical measures of our physical performance: How much oxygen we can take in, how efficiently blood is pumped through the system to deliver this oxygen, and how well oxygen is utilized by the muscles and other cells of the body constitute a strong measure of fitness. Even though aging brings about a natural decline in these areas, a sedentary lifestyle will cause significant acceleration. The changes we all experience due to passage of time alone have much less impact than those we inflict on ourselves by the way we live.

The lungs have an amazing surface area to cater to our continuous need for oxygen. If lung tissue were spread out, it would cover almost half a tennis court. Healthy lungs can hold between 4 and 6 quarts of air, and we can sustain muscular work for hours without stopping because of this tremendous lung capacity. But we have to breathe in large amounts of air to get the oxygen we need, and during strenuous exercise such as running there is a dramatic increase in air intake, heart rate, and blood flow. There is a great increase in the volume of blood brought to active muscles, and blood is diverted from inactive areas, such as the digestive system, to support the working muscles. Deeper breathing during demanding exercise causes a tremendous increase in the amount of air brought into the lungs. The number of breaths per minute increases, and the volume of air we take in with each breath rises considerably. More oxygen is extracted from the air we breathe in, and there is a considerable rise in the volume of oxygen taken up by the working muscles. This greatly increased breathing rate during exercise does more than increase oxygen supply. It also helps to cool the system, just as sweating does. We lose heat all the time through breathing, and the faster we breathe, the more heat we lose. But only if the cardiorespiratory system is in a good state of health can all these functions take place efficiently.

Just as a car engine cannot fire on all cylinders unless gasoline combines freely with oxygen, the body cannot function without enough oxygen. If a chronic lung condition is present, the ability to take in or expel oxygen is greatly affected, setting limits in daily living and during exercise. Two of these chronic conditions should be briefly discussed to understand the limitations with which some participants might be confronted.

chronic bronchitis

Chronic bronchitis is a disabling disease caused by persistent irritation of the bronchi. Heavy smoking is the most common irritant and the major cause of this disease, and air pollutants also play a role. The smoker's cough is evidence of inflammation in the bronchi, and the mucus coughed up by a smoker is a sign of damage to the cilia, the fine hairs that line the entire respiratory tract. The combination of excess mucus and damaged cilia impairs drainage and promotes bacterial growth. Breathing becomes progressively harder as the bronchi become narrow and lung tissue is destroyed. Those with severe bronchitis cannot walk very far or climb stairs without experiencing extreme shortness of breath and will be limited in their ability to participate in activity.

emphysema

Emphysema tends to be associated with a long history of chronic bronchitis. It causes air sacs to overinflate and occasionally rupture, and the person suffering from emphysema experiences great difficulty in expelling air. "Many patients with emphysema also have an asthmatic component to their condition," explained Dr. Peterman. "Bronchial tubes tend to be dynamic, and a patient with emphysema can have asthmatic triggers, and exercise can be one of these triggers. This means that exercise can induce asthma and make it worse unless it is prevented by using an inhaler before exercise participation. Exercise-induced asthma should not necessarily prevent people from being active, but they need to be medically advised and often rely on medication."

Emphysema, once it exists, is irreversible and tends to get progressively worse unless contributing habits are stopped. Daily living can become a constant struggle for necessary oxygen, and persons so seriously afflicted are not likely to participate in our programs. If the condition is less severe and allows exercise, the person will obviously be limited and needs to participate within these limits. "Emphysema is not made worse by exercising," Dr. Peterman explained. "I need to say again that sensible exercise within the person's given limitation, no matter what the condition, should be a normal part of daily living, and you are always better off by including it in your life. But it needs to be understood and respected that a person suffering from a chronic lung condition will have markedly reduced capacity. They can participate, but at a low level because they simply don't have the oxygen supply available to work beyond a certain limit."

"I encourage patients to get out and walk to get their circulation moving. The lung damage is there to stay—exercise can make no change there. But exercise will improve the condition of their muscles and develop greater efficiency in the use and distribution of oxygen to the periphery, a very important factor in these conditions. These clearly are self-limiting conditions, and there will be self-selection when it comes to exercise participation. The people who will join a program feel capable of doing a certain amount, and they will make good decisions based on what they experience. Unless a patient has a variant of emphysema with a strong asthmatic component to exercise, they won't hurt themselves in reasonable activity. In fact, it is desirable from a medical standpoint that they do all they can to improve their overall physical condition within the limits set by their problem."

dizziness

A number of participants in my program experience occasional dizziness during exercise. Dizziness can be brought on by a variety of causes. An inner ear problem may cause what is called "positional vertigo," which can be triggered by certain positions. Vertigo makes everything spin and can make the person very nauseous. "Vertigo is usually easy to tell apart from other kinds of dizziness," explained Dr. Peterman, "and it can generally be prevented by avoiding the position which may bring it on."

"Then there is the experience of light-headedness, causing a person to feel that they may faint. There are many older persons who can bring this on by hyperextending the neck—as in looking up at the ceiling, for example. This can actually impinge on the blood supply to the brain, leaving the brain with too little oxygen. Again, avoiding these movements should prevent this light-headedness from occurring. Low blood pressure may be another cause because inadequate blood supply reaches the brain."

"Sometimes dizziness occurs on straightening up from forward bending, or after a person has been kneeling for a while and then stands up. While kneeling, leg muscles tighten up and there is no pooling of blood. But on standing, the muscles are no longer under stress and blood will pool in the legs, again limiting blood supply to the brain. If a person is in very poor physical condition, blood vessels are not used to having to react to changes in position. But the efficiency of blood vessels to adapt can be improved by regular exposure to physical movement and changes in position, so I believe that here, too, exercise can bring positive changes. A good example may be the person who has been confined to bed for a prolonged period after surgery. When we first get this person out of bed in the hospital, they are often very, very dizzy. After lying down for so long doing nothing, their system just can't handle this upright posture. We then have to use a tilt table in physical therapy and gradually tilt the patient up, longer and more often each day, until the blood vessels learn to adapt again. In terms of people with these problems participating in exercise, I would expect these same improvements."

Heat and humidity may be a factor, causing overexertion during exercise. Nausea may also be the result of having come to class without breakfast, creating low blood sugar and leaving the person with too little energy for the activity. Encourage participants not to skip breakfast, especially not when they know that an active hour is ahead.

If someone experiences dizziness or vertigo, take action quickly. The best position for this person is to lie flat on the floor with legs elevated on a chair so that blood flow is quickly diverted from the lower extremities to the brain. They feel better quickly. Within 5 to 10 minutes, they can slowly come to a sitting position, stay put for a while to make sure that they feel all right, and then sit on a chair for a while and not participate again until they feel well enough to do so. Should something like this occur during the class hour, it is important to stay calm and deal with the situation appropriately. It may be necessary to have participants stop their activities for the time it takes you to help, but take care to keep panic from breaking out in the classroom. A sense of humor helps once you have established that the person is not in real distress, and you can return to teaching while the person is resting.

depression

Much has been said and written about the close relationship between mental and physical well-being. A healthy mind helps the body keep its vigor, and an active body supports a positive mental attitude. If we keep mental and physical challenges in our lives, we develop confidence in ourselves, and this confidence makes it easier to seek out and meet new challenges. If we continue being receptive to new experiences, our lives will be enriched. These basic facts do not change as we age; living a full and interesting life is not a privilege of the young. Doors to new involvements and experiences can be opened at any age, and retirement can present us with the time we may not have had before to explore new options.

One of my students called me to rejoin our class again after having been away. "I have to make sure to keep time in my schedule for exercise because my calendar is filling up fast," she said. She had just signed up for two college courses and had organized a book discussion group for seniors to meet regularly at her home. In addition, she is spending several hours a day with her professional work as a writer. Madeline is 80 years old, and when I responded to her busy calendar by saying, "It sounds like you won't have much opportunity to be bored," she replied that boredom is something she would never allow herself to experience. "There are too many things to do and tackle to sit around bored or depressed," she said. "Life is too short for that!"

"Of all the reasons I can think of to encourage people into activity, depression would be a major one," said Dr. Peterman. "Depression is a common and serious problem among the elderly patients I see, and it affects the quality of their daily lives so much." The social causes of depression among the elderly are nearly always associated with separation and loss. The retirement process, for many, is a period of great stress. Life changes drastically, and if work has been a major source of satisfaction and purpose, being without it leaves a great void. Children marry and move away, causing another major change. The loss of a spouse and the adjustment to living alone is the most dramatic and difficult experience. In addition, friends may become incapacitated or die, making the older person's support system smaller and smaller.

It is also a fact that our culture does not make the older generation feel valued and important. Grappling with this new stage in life can become an overwhelming task that requires finding new inner resources and developing new coping skills and may result in isolation and depression. "But I firmly believe," Dr. Peterman said, "that one can come out of these difficult changes with a feeling of vitality rather than feeling that we have lost our handle on life. There is another life out there in spite of all that may have happened. Isolation is a self-perpetuating problem unless there is intervention, and I am a firm believer in exercise as being one of the most important forms of intervention at any age. Feeling in control of your body, getting out, feeling good about yourself because you are exercising, and feeling better physically has a direct effect on mental well-being. It's no different for the older person than for someone younger. Activity is a wonderful tonic. Avoiding isolation and depression should be one of the best reasons for older people to become involved in exercise programs."

"Bringing many of these isolated people in contact with each other in such exercise programs is a great thing," Dr. Peterman went on to say. "I am quite convinced that if more older people would actively participate in these organized programs, we as physicians would see much less depression and less use of medication to deal with this problem. I would so much rather use natural ways of dealing with depression than having patients resort to medication. It's easiest to write a prescription and hand it to a patient, and unfortunately that's what most patients want. It's the easy way out. You don't have to make an effort and apply yourself to making your life more meaningful if a pill can make you feel better. But I believe that what makes a person really feel well again is to take action, to take life into his or her own hands and do something good with it. So I am conservative when it comes to medication in general and instead try to help my patients look at their options and choices. I obviously feel this way in regard to all the conditions we have discussed, and depression is no exception."

Sadness is probably the most common sign of depression. People who are chronically depressed always look sad; their faces are immobile, and they show little emotion. They rarely smile and can spend much time gazing into space, looking as if they are about to burst into tears. Crying can become a habit, and many depressed people cry a lot, most often when they are alone. There may be sleep disturbances, appetite loss, neglect of appearance, anxiety, indecision, tiredness, weakness, and poor concentration. If someone in your program appears sad over a period of time, it may be of great help and support to them if you create an opportunity for a quiet, caring conversation. Just knowing that you have noticed the sadness and are concerned may lift his or her spirits. Additional help and advice may come from counseling or medical intervention, and you may be instrumental in encouraging the person to seek such help and support during this difficult time. Give strong encouragement for staying with your program, even if there seems little noticeable enthusiasm in participation. Our programs should not only serve our older students' need for physical exercise. They also can be reliable support during times of change and crisis.

12
nutrition
in the
later years

Not very much is known abut the nutrient requirements of the elderly. Guidelines have been established
for pregnancy, infancy, adolescence, and adult men and
women. The Recommended Dietary Allowances (RDA)
provide standards for the U.S. on desirable levels of
nutrient intakes that are high enough to protect us
against dietary deficiencies. For adults, these standards
are presented in only two categories, 25-50 years and
51 years and above, despite the obvious criticism that a
person of 90 is unlikely to have the same nutrient
needs as a person at 51. No adequate nationwide study
has been conducted of the nutritional well-being of older
Americans. Nor is there, at this time, a data base for
making specific recommendations for those over 65.
Any recommendations that are made are based on a
combination of experimental results, clinical experience,
and logical deduction and have to be considered
tentative.

One problem with studies that have been conducted is that they have been cross-sectional. What is
not known now is which changes take place within a
given individual over a lifetime of certain nutritional
habits. Studies that have compared elderly subjects
with young subjects give inadequate information. The
federal government, however, has recently invested $30
million to establish the Human Nutrition Research
Center on Aging at Tufts University, the world's first
research center of its kind. There, basic research on
nutrition will be combined with specific investigations of
some conditions of aging that appear to be caused, or
that might be prevented, by a change in eating habits.
When it is in full operation, the center will become
home to more than 200 resident researchers and staff
members, up to 28 elderly volunteer residents, and as
many as 15,000 old mice, rats, and rabbits. Research
will be funded by the Department of Agriculture, and

this massive investment is needed because, after a hundred years of scientific medicine, no one has answers to frustrating questions relating to diet and aging. The challenge facing the investigators will consist of identifying conditions of diet and lifestyle that best preserve bodily functions while minimizing the development of degenerative disease.

Professor Virginia Beal of the University of Massachusetts has been in the field of nutrition for 40 years and has been witness to many changes and developments over this period of time. Professor Beal is author of *Nutrition in the Lifespan*, a widely used text for university-level nutrition courses. Spending time with Professor Beal in preparation for this nutrition chapter has been very informative, and I am grateful for her willingness to share her knowledge and answer many of my questions patiently and thoroughly.

Exercise physiologists, medical researchers, and nutritionists have been able to determine certain biological changes that are a normal part of the aging process, and it is accepted that the rate of change differs from one person to the next depending on genetic predisposition, lifestyle, and health status. The body becomes less efficient in many different ways. Metabolism slows by an estimated 15% between the ages of 30 and 80. There is a significant decrease in energy requirement (caloric needs). Oxygen uptake and utilization become less efficient. There is loss of lean body mass, mostly due to the wasting of muscle and an increase in the ratio of fat tissue to lean tissue. The gastrointestinal tract through which all food must pass to be absorbed and digested undergoes progressive changes, as do the kidneys, which must excrete the waste products of the foods we digest. Basically, all cells in the body are affected by aging, requiring some alterations in the amount and kinds of foods we ingest.

caloric needs

The only clear age-related recommendation that has been made relates to the need for reducing calorie intake. Because physiological functions decline and we are much less active as we age, we no longer can afford to eat as much as we used to when we were younger. Professor Hamish Munro of the Massachusetts Institute of Technology has conducted cross-sectional studies and provides data showing a progressive reduction in total energy intake from 2,700 kcal at age 30 to 2,100 kcal at age 80 among the groups of men he studied. This difference of 600 kcal daily represents a 200 kcal reduction due to lowered metabolism and a significant 400 kcal reduction resulting from greatly decreased levels of physical activity. "This is one area no one has studied very much," Professor Beal points

out. "How do caloric needs change in people who continue to stay very active throughout life and into the older years? It's one of the many questions we don't have the answers to at this time."

Professor Beal feels that the above figures for caloric intake seem quite high and that there are few older persons who can afford to consume 2,000 daily calories without putting on unwanted pounds. She points to studies that indicate that free-living, relatively active older women volunteering as subjects generally consume somewhere around 1,300 to 1,400 kcal. This is below the RDA recommendations of an average of 1,600 kcal, with a range from 1,200 to 2,000 kcal. "One problem with the need for caloric restriction at an older age is that there is every indication that the body still has the same requirements for protein, minerals, and vitamins. In fact, some needs may be greater simply because the body is less efficient in absorbing and utilizing these important nutrients," explains Professor Beal. "We are less efficient in digesting food and absorbing nutrients across the intestinal wall. The cells are slower in function, which means that nutrients are absorbed less efficiently. Intake, absorption, and utilization all change so that we have a number of important factors to consider, both in getting food to the system and then having the body use it."

With some quick calculations, however, Professor Beal arrives at the reassuring fact that it is quite possible to meet the recommended nutrient requirements with a carefully chosen diet—there just isn't much room for the "empty calories" younger persons can indulge in. Caloric needs vary with age, sex, and activity, but we share the need to balance caloric intake with energy output from physical activity to control weight. If physical activity is greatly reduced, fewer calories are needed, but it is important to keep good variety and nutritional balance in the daily diet, and it helps greatly to be informed about some nutrition basics.

Proteins, carbohydrates, and fats are essential nutrients that provide calories. Proteins and carbohydrates provide 4 calories per gram of food weight, while fats provide 9 calories per gram. "Refined carbohydrates and fats are where reductions need to be made so that a nutritionally balanced diet can be maintained given the lowered caloric needs of an older person," explains Professor Beal. "Foods have to be selected more carefully, but it is certainly possible to keep good variety in the daily diet and have meals be an enjoyable part of life."

carbohydrates

It is important to understand some basics about carbohydrates. For many people today, carbohydrates like bread and potatoes are considered to be the calorie villains in any diet attempt. Dr. Jean Mayer, respected for his work in human nutrition, once conducted a survey of people's beliefs about bread. He found that people of all ages and economic backgrounds grossly overestimated the calorie content of bread and that it is usually the first food to disappear from the table of the weight-conscious and is replaced by more protein. Yet the simple fact is that there is absolutely no difference in calories between carbohydrates and proteins: Each provide 4 calories per gram.

Ignorance causes us to go along with popular beliefs, and most of us know too little about these mysterious carbohydrates. It's confusing to learn that foods as dissimilar as lima beans, alcohol, grapefruit, candy bars, and milk all are carbohydrate foods.

There are simple, complex, and refined carbohydrates. Even the crunch in celery is caused by a carbohydrate: cellulose, a no-calorie fiber. The many different forms of carbohydrates vary greatly in nutritional quality and calories; some are very fattening without having any other nutrients whatsoever. It is interesting to look at these different categories more closely to know what contributions they make (or often don't make) to our daily diet.

Complex carbohydrates are the "good guys," the foods that provide us with vitamins, minerals, and fibers. They are found in whole grains, vegetables, fruits, and legumes. The body must break down a long chain of molecules to convert complex carbohydrates into blood sugar, or glucose, which is used for energy. Calories from these good foods are released slowly and evenly over an extended period of time and keep us satisfied.

Simple carbohydrates, or sugars, are found naturally occurring in fruits, vegetables, milk, and honey. Refined, they come to us as table sugar, syrups, cakes, candy, and soda pop. Simple carbohydrates are absorbed very quickly because their molecules are smaller and will bring blood sugar levels into high gear for short periods. Most refined carbohydrates provide no other nutrients but plenty of calories. "Even honey which is so promoted has essentially no other nutrients," Professor Beal points out. "And the body's ability to process sugars decreases with aging along with the general decrease in glandular function. If the pancreas is not as efficient as it used to be, it's probably not releasing enough insulin to deal with the large amounts of sugar contained in refined carbohydrates. If body cells are somewhat less efficient in removing glucose from the

blood, there will be higher blood sugar levels especially for persons with certain health problems such as diabetes. It certainly is far preferable to get the calories and nutrients we need from complex, wholesome carbohydrates."

Refined carbohyrates are created by our food industry. Most minerals, vitamins, and fiber are stripped from whole foods in refining and processing to produce convenient, packageable foods with long shelf life. Examples of refining are the removal of bran and wheat germ from grains to turn them into white flour or the polishing of brown rice to make it white and fluffy. Processed foods tend to be expensive and are a poor nutritional bargain.

Alcohol is not a true carbohydrate but is made from carbohydrate foods. It tends to be a source of "empty calories" and adds about 250 calories per day to the average diet of drinking-age Americans.

Fiber, too, is in the carbohydrate family. We know fiber as "bulk" or "roughage" and know that it is important in the passage of food. Fiber has no calories and is not absorbed by the human body because it is indigestible, but it is a very important part of our diet and will be discussed later in this chapter.

Carbohydrates are the major source of energy for the human body. They are the only true "brain food," as Dr. Mayer puts it. Carbohydrates are essential for everyone, despite their poor and confusing reputation. We even need them for efficient metabolism of fats we eat.

Three of every five calories Americans now eat come from fats and sugars. Processed foods make up more than half of what we eat, and consumption of whole grains and potatoes has gone down considerably over the years. So many nutritionally empty fat and sugar calories are eaten that it is quite possible to be overweight and yet undernourished. The U.S. Dietary Goals strongly recommend an increase in our present low intake of complex carbohydrates from 28% of our daily calories to 48%. Simple carbohydrates should be reduced from the present 18% of our daily calories to 10% at most. Unfortunately, processed and refined foods are what appeal most to a large percentage of the population: soft bread, white rice, puffed and heavily sugared cereals, crackers, potato chips, candy bars, and donuts. These tend to be nonnutritious, loaded with calories, and therefore fattening. They replace carbohydrates such as baked potatoes, oatmeal, whole grain breads, apples and carrots, and fresh fruit juices—all the natural, healthful foods that also provide other nutrients.

The problem is not that carbohydrates are fattening, but that we make poor food choices. And for many of us, it isn't even a matter of ignorance; we choose poorly in spite of being informed and knowing better. Fortunately, it's never too late to make positive changes, and improvements in the carbohydrate area of our daily diet are easy to come by. Eating more fresh fruits and vegetables means getting bulk in the form of no-calorie fibers. Hot oatmeal in the morning instead of lining up cereal boxes will provide a nutritious, satisfying breakfast. No one but the food industry benefits from starting our day with snaps, crackles, and pops. We can take advantage of choice fresh vegetables and fruits at farm stands and in supermarkets. And we can be more conscious of reducing the sugars in our diet. Sugar is hidden in many processed foods, even salty ones such as bacon, canned soups, salad dressings, and TV dinners. Those who are concerned about weight should be equally concerned about good health when deciding to eliminate certain foods from the diet. Help your students to make good choices by sharing some of this information.

proteins

In the human body, proteins make up three fourths of all the solid matter. Every cell in the body contains some protein. Protein is part of muscle, bone, cartilage, skin, and blood. There are four basic kinds of proteins. *Structural* proteins are part of bones, skin, and nails. *Contractile* proteins, which can lengthen and shorten, enable our muscles to function so that we can move around, and they aid internal contractions like swallowing, heart beats, and breathing. The *transport* proteins carry oxygen and nutrients in the blood and deliver these needed materials to all cells. The last group is known as *process-activating* proteins, which the body breaks down into amino acids needed for construction. It is not clearly known how the body breaks down the foods we take in, but most of the work is done by enzymes that are produced by the hundreds in each cell.

Protein intake is of vital importance in our daily diet so that all the millions of bodily chemical processes can take place. With protein, the body forms new cells and repairs worn-out ones, transports nutrients into and out of cells, and regulates the balance of water and acids. Protein is needed to make antibodies that help us fight infection and is essential to the clotting of blood and formation of scar tissue. The protein in blood vessels is elastic, allowing them to expand and contract to maintain normal blood pressure. All enzymes and many hormones are proteins.

Even though all bodily functions depend on protein, we don't need very much of it in our daily diet. The notion that athletic activity or strenuous exercise demands extra protein is a myth, and similarly false is the idea that everyone must consume large amounts of protein to build muscles and stay healthy. Most adults need a

relatively small proportion of their daily food intake in the form of proteins: Only about 10 to 15% of calories should come from protein. Americans are protein-consumers, eating far more than people in other parts of the world and certainly more than is needed by the body. Eight amino acids that adults need have to be provided by dietary protein because the body cannot manufacture them, and they have to be provided in adequate quantities. If even one of these essential amino acids is lacking in the diet for only a short time, its absence limits the production of proteins in the body. The "complete" proteins, which contain all eight of these essential amino acids in about the right proportions, are found mainly in animal foods: meats, eggs, and dairy products. Most vegetable proteins are deficient in one or more of the essential amino acids. Combining two or more plant foods or adding small quantities of animal products to an incomplete plant protein source can combine into the complete protein the body needs.

High-protein consumption can make us fat because the most common sources of protein in our diet—meat and dairy products—are high in fat and calories, contributing to the problems of cholesterol and obesity. For many persons, excess protein consumption can also create problems in the form of excess nitrogen, which is contained in protein foods and needs to be excreted by the kidneys. "Carbohydrates and fats are made up of carbon, hydrogen, and oxygen, and the body can dispose of these very easily when they finally break down into carbon dioxide and water. But the nitrogen contained in protein has to be disposed of through the kidneys, and this presents a problem for people with kidney disease. For older persons in general, protein intake should not exceed what is needed by the body because kidney function and efficiency decline with age. Low-protein diets are prescribed if kidney disease is present to take this additional strain away from damaged kidneys," explains Professor Beal.

"Investigations indicate that there is little change in protein requirements from early adulthood to old age, even though body mass, and especially muscle mass, decreases. But there may very well be a need for more protein rather than less as we age. Stop to consider that every cell in the body requires protein, that all the enzymes, hormones, and most of the body materials are made up of protein, and that the cell structure itself is basically protein. In order for a cell to reproduce, it has to have the amino acids from protein to make the new cell. And if we become less efficient in doing this as we get older, we need to be sure that we get enough and probably more than enough in order for the body to get what it needs. High-protein foods also are concentrated sources of important minerals and vitamins, and when caloric intake becomes more restricted, we need to look at how to get the most nutrients out of the foods we eat. I realize that an opposing picture presents itself here—on the one hand we say that too much protein can strain an older person's kidneys, and on the other hand it appears that the need for protein may increase to provide the body with enough. But in the absence of kidney disease, a diet in which 10 to 15% of the daily calories come from protein seems well tolerated and protects against depletion of trace minerals."

It is interesting to look at protein concentration in different foods to understand which are good sources. Our own bodies are largely water, and so are those of other animals. Therefore, the protein content of meat, fish, and poultry after cooking is no more than 20 to 30%. Lean meats have more protein per pound, and fatter meats and oily fish have less. This, ironically, means that "prime" cuts contain less protein than tougher, less expensive grades of meat and, of course, are much higher in fat.

Protein is quite concentrated in most cheeses. Harder, more compact cheeses tend to be more protein-rich than softer or runnier cheeses. Cheddar is about 25% protein by weight, whereas cottage cheese may have only half as much. Processed cheeses are somewhere in between.

In terms of the quality and wide range of amino acids in their protein, eggs are unsurpassed. But protein density is only about 13%, about the same as the lowest protein cottage cheese.

When looking at vegetables, nuts are at the top of the list, averaging about 15 to 16% protein. Grain products are next at between 8 and 9%. Most breakfast cereals, made from grains, are in this range. But the protein of these foods is incomplete unless several plant proteins are combined or supplemented with small amounts of cheese or meat. Legumes (dry peas and beans) have a protein concentration of between 4 and 6%. And the figures go down to between 2 to 3% for most other fruits and vegetables.

A basic, simple rule is used to determine how much protein adults need, and the requirement is essentially the same for men as for women. Because food composition tables give protein in grams, it is the measure used. The Food and Nutrition Board recommendation is for .424 grams of protein needed for each pound of body weight. For the person weighing 140 pounds, for example, this would mean around 60 grams of protein daily.

Nutritionists recommend that a well-balanced diet should derive a third of its protein from animal sources and two thirds from plant sources. Legumes are the richest sources of vegetable protein, and when combined with rice or grains, provide a healthy, low-fat meal. In comparison, many animal proteins contain more fat than protein. In a T-bone steak, about 20% of the calories are protein; the remaining 80% are fat calories. In hard cheeses, only a quarter of the calories come from protein; the rest is fat. Whole milk offers protein at 21% of the calories, and fat provides 48%. Chicken without skin is a "skinny" protein source with only 31% fat and 64% protein calories.

Table 12.1 is a short list of protein sources, taken from *Jane Brody's Nutrition Book*. Published in 1981, it is now available in paperback and is a wonderful source of down-to-earth, factual nutrition information for the lay reader.

Table 12.1 Sources of Protein

Protein Source	Serving	Calories
Chicken without skin, roasted	2.2 oz	114
Cod, broiled	2.2 oz	107
Pork, lean only	2.1 oz	162
Boiled ham	3.3 oz	220
Frankfurter	3 franks	456
Egg, boiled or poached	3 eggs	240
American cheese	2.7 oz	288
Milk, whole	17.5 oz	338
Milk, skimmed	17.5 oz	180
Peanut butter	4.5 tbsp	422
Tuna in oil, drained	2.2 oz	122
Sirloin, regular, broiled	2.7 oz	300
Sirloin, lean only, broiled	2.0 oz	115

Note. From *Jane Brody's Nutrition Book* (p. 46) by Jane Brody, 1981, New York: W.W. Norton & Company. Reprinted with permission.

fats

No recommended allowances have been established for fat in the diet, but we don't need to be concerned about not getting enough. The problem for most of us is that we get too much.

Beyond providing energy, fats serve many useful functions. In the body, fat cushions organs, forms an energy storage depot under the skin and keeps heat from escaping too fast. Fats carry vitamins A, D, E, and K. One part of fat, linoleic acid, is an essential nutrient that cannot be manufactured by the body and is vital for normal growth and healthy skin. Fortunately, it is present in many kinds of foods and is especially abundant in vegetable oils, some nuts, and poultry. Fats are digested slowly and contribute to the pleasant feelings of fullness. Fats also make foods taste good.

The body's needs for the various functions of fat can be met by a daily diet containing 15 to 25 grams, according to the RDA committee, and linoleic acid should be 1 to 2% of caloric intake. This means that 1 to 2 tablespoons of fat daily are adequate, and some of this intake needs to be in the form of unsaturated fats. All dietary fats have some combination of saturated and unsaturated fatty acids, and the ratio depends mainly on whether the fat is of animal or vegetable origin. Foods from animal sources, such as meat, butter, milk, cheese, and eggs are high in saturated fats, which are usually solid at room temperature, but also contain unsaturated fats. Vegetable oils or margarine, in comparison, are high in polyunsaturated fats, which are generally liquid at room temperature. (The percentages and mixtures of fats are different in each food.) Even though many food sources of fats are obvious, some are not, at least not visibly: Pecan nuts, for example, are 70% to 80% fat. Similarly rich in fats are many processed foods, including baked goods and chocolate.

The saturated fats get most of the blame as researchers look at the relationship between heart and blood vessel disease and high-fat diets. Unsaturated fats are believed to do much less harm to arteries, but all fats have been implicated in contributing to some types of cancer. Concern about high fat intake is very real: In the average American diet, fats provide 40 to 55% of total daily calories, and that is too much for good health. Of this intake, saturated fats supply 16%, monounsaturated fats 19%, and polyunsaturated fats 7% of total calories. The U.S. Dietary Goals recommend a decrease of total fat to 30% of daily calories, equally divided into saturated, monounsaturated, and polyunsaturated fats.

"There is no evidence that requirements for essential fatty acids change with age. But tolerance to fat may be reduced in some people, and certain health problems may require limited fat consumption. Sound nutritional advice would be to cut down on fat intake in general and concentrate on more nutritious sources of calories. Fat is fattening at 100 calories per tablespoon—whether it is unsaturated or saturated, whether it is margarine, butter, oil, or meat fat. Because we need relatively little for bodily functions, it is wise to reduce our fat intake and enjoy other, more healthful foods instead," Professor Beal suggests.

fiber

Even though adequate fiber intake is important for digestion, there are some disadvantages to be aware of, according to Professor Beal, especially when making recommendations to an older population. It has been shown that people who have a very high fiber intake have a decrease in the absorption of important minerals, which go through the system and are not picked up. Especially for the older person who already has a lower nutrient absorption in general, this lowered min-

eral absorption can create problems. "We are now seriously looking at the fact that older people may need more minerals than the RDA suggests. There already has been an increase in the figures suggested for calcium requirements, for example. Zinc is another mineral being investigated, and recommendations for zinc requirements will probably be increased before long, too. The science of nutrition is relatively new, and there will continue to be changes in recommendations."

Constipation, a problem for many older persons, can be greatly relieved if adequate fiber is contained in the daily diet. In addition, there is a direct relationship between muscular function and digestive problems because the passage of food is dependent on action of muscles all the way along the intestinal tract. "Activity is a significant contributor to eliminating problems with constipation," Professor Beal emphasizes. "There has been general appreciation of the fact that people who exercise regularly experience far fewer problems with colon function, and this is important to educate older persons about. In addition, fluid intake is something to keep in mind because fluids keep the contents of the gastrointestinal tract soft and make passage of food easier. So we have the combination of fiber, exercise, and fluids as preventive measures, rather than resorting to laxatives, which, unfortunately, many older people do."

Mineral oil is one laxative agent that should definitely be avoided. Mineral oil absorbs fat-soluble vitamins, making them unavailable to the body. In general, Professor Beal believes that many people become addicted to laxatives. "If maybe only psychologically—but they come to think that they simply can't have a bowel movement without laxatives. But if roughage and fluids in the diet are adequate and regular exercise is adhered to, there should be no need for laxatives. It's not normal to need them, and not healthy to use them."

fluid intake

Some concern has recently been expressed about inadequate fluid intake among the elderly population. The January 1985 issue of the *Tufts University Diet and Nutrition Letter* carried a report entitled "Aging and Thirst: A Not to Be Overlooked Connection." The report stated that new findings indicate that elderly people may not necessarily feel thirsty when their bodies are in need of fluid and, therefore, may run the risk of dehydration. British researchers compared the effects of lack of water in a group of healthy men between the ages of 67 and 75 to those in men under the age of 32. After a full day of ingesting a diet of dry foods and no beverages, the older men felt significantly less thirsty than the younger men, even though both groups lost about the same amount of body fluid. And when the men were allowed to drink water without limit, the older men drank less than half the volume consumed by the younger subjects.

The feeling of thirst is triggered when inadequate fluid intake lowers blood levels of water and sodium becomes more concentrated in the blood stream. But the above study showed that the older group of subjects experienced "a remarkable lack of thirst and discomfort" compared to the younger men and did not drink enough water to restore their blood to normal. The older subjects' kidneys did not hold onto water as would have been expected to compensate for the fluid deprivation. "This study suggests that, as you age, the body is less likely to tell you when it needs water. Thus, to meet the essential need of about 6 to 8 cups a day—be it from water itself or any beverage—it's a good idea to get into the habit of drinking something with each meal or between meals, even if you don't feel the urge. Indeed, it's difficult to drink too much water," the report recommends.

When I discuss fluid intake with class members, there is general agreement that they experience less thirst and drink little during the course of a day, especially water. I have made it a habit to bring gallon containers of clean, good-tasting well water to my classes and encourage everyone to drink before, during, and after exercise. Making participants aware of being more concerned about adequate fluid intake during exercise has helped them make changes in their drinking habits in general.

vitamins and minerals

Because vitamins do not contain calories, they do not provide energy. Neither do they contribute any material to tissue building. But vitamins are indispensable catalysts to assist enzymes in turning nutrients into energy and body tissues. Vitamins and enzymes help a chemical process get started and control its speed. The amounts of vitamins required daily are so small that they are specified in milligrams or micrograms.

Four vitamins (A, D, E, and K) are soluble in fat and insoluble in water. They usually enter the body with fatty foods, are stored in body fat and in the liver in small quantities when not needed, and therefore do not have to be included in each day's meals. The other nine vitamins (vitamin C plus eight of the B-vitamin family) dissolve in water and are not stored in the body. Any surplus is excreted in the urine. Because they are not stored, these water soluble vitamins should be included in each day's food intake in adequate amounts.

By the end of the 17th century, many ships' surgeons recognized that the lack of fresh fruits and vegetables on long voyages led to scurvy, a debilitating and often fatal disease. By 1753, The British physician James Lind proved with a controlled experiment that people could avoid scurvy by drinking citrus juices. But it was not until 1928 that vitamin C was isolated and recognized as the crucial scurvy preventive. Since then, the biochemical roles of 13 vitamins have been identified, and vitamin deficiency diseases such as pellegra, scurvy, and beriberi are now rare.

Most nutrition authorities maintain that the average person in this country gets more than enough of the essential nutrients simply by eating a good variety of common foods. Very few people in the industrialized world suffer from deficiencies. Most vitamins and minerals occur in many foods. Many other foods (such as cereals, milk, and margarine) are artificially enriched with many vitamins and minerals.

But with increasing age, the levels of vitamins in the body tend to fall, even among people eating a good diet. Illness can upset the body's vitamin-using processes, and medical treatments can block the absorption of certain vitamins and minerals. Chronic use of laxatives, antibiotics, oral diabetic drugs, and some anti-inflammatory drugs can cause depletion of certain vitamins and minerals. Lowered caloric intake brings in fewer nutrients in general, and tight food budgets are a reality for many elderly. Some avoid certain major food groups (milk products, fresh fruits and vegetables) due to health reasons or food preference, and low blood levels of certain nutrients are found in many elderly persons.

Professor Beal points out that those elderly especially prone to marginal deficiencies tend to live alone with some degree of physical disability which prevents them from going out to purchase fresh foods of a good variety regularly. Loneliness and depression may result in poor eating habits and little interest in fixing meals. "Even though I am opposed to vitamin supplements in general, people under certain circumstances do benefit, and a well-balanced, one-a-day vitamin certainly can do no harm. It is always preferable to get the nutrients, minerals, and vitamins we need from our foods—but in some situations, supplementation is important for health."

Despite tight food budgets, many elderly fall prey to costly nutritional quackery: the promises of better health, lasting youthfulness, and greater longevity in the form of "health foods" and special supplements loaded with megadoses of various vitamins and minerals. But, according to Professor Beal, "Megadoses of any kind may be harmful to the elderly or anyone else. Elderly people are more susceptible to the sales tactics used by these industries. They promise magical cures, the fountain of youth, and life extension—and who wouldn't want all those things at that age? Sales people even come to the door and can use sales approaches which are very effective with an older population. What I am concerned about is the fact that these sales people often were selling shoes the week before and tend to have absolutely no scientifically based nutrition knowledge. Their job is to sell a product, and they work very hard at their sales pitches."

Those who succumb to these pressures and promises may spend $30 monthly on a variety of supplements, with bottles of pills, powders, and liquids lined up for "self-medication," something Professor Beal and colleagues in her field are quite concerned about. "The average person has little nutrition knowledge and no understanding of how nutrients need to be balanced to be absorbed and utilized by the body. People take single nutrients in megadoses without in any way understanding their effects, and that is very dangerous. We worry about toxic reactions to fat-soluble vitamins, which stay in the system and can accumulate. We are less concerned about the water-soluble vitamins because the body can rid itself of excesses. But it is not a good idea to take any single nutrient supplement, especially in the megadose quantities, which are so popular. Vitamins and minerals have no magical powers, cannot cure diseases other than those caused by deficiencies, cannot keep us young, or make us live longer. Those who take supplements should stay with a multipurpose, one-a-day supplement that comes close to the RDA recommendations—the vitamins and minerals contained in these are scientifically balanced so that the body can better utilize them. And don't let pill-taking lull you into thinking that you can afford to skimp on the variety and quality of your daily food intake. Keep wholesome, nutritious foods in your diet—they are the best source of all nutrients you need. Supplements are a little added insurance, not a substitute for food."

minerals

Minerals, too, have become big business since the field of vitamins has proved so fertile. Shelves of health food stores are stocked with bottles of calcium, magnesium, zinc, iron, dolomite, potassium chloride, and the rest. But we can receive adequate amounts of both major and trace minerals from the foods we eat without these expensive bottled supplies. Whether it be of animal or vegetable origin, all food comes to us from either soil or sea. The chemical composition of soil or water depends on the rocks that lie beneath them and are composed of complex mineral salts containing a variety of major minerals and trace elements. The major minerals (magnesium, calcium, sodium, and potassium) are contained in considerable quantities in our food. Trace minerals, also called trace elements, include iron, zinc, selenium, manganese, copper, iodine, chromium,

and fluorine. Our foods contain these in much smaller amounts, and the body needs only small quantities.

The role of minerals in the body is extremely varied, and that of some trace minerals not completely understood. It is known that fluorine helps prevent tooth decay, but the part manganese plays has not been established. Iodine is essential for the normal functioning of the thyroid gland. When not enough iodine is present in the diet, the gland enlarges into what is called a goiter, which can interfere with speech and breathing. Goiter was once prevalent in the midwestern states but has been eliminated, along with other deficiency diseases, by adding essential vitamins and minerals to common foods. Most salt we buy contains iodine. Vitamin D is added to milk to prevent rickets, a bone-deforming disease in children. White bread contains added niacin, which prevents pellegra; thiamin, which prevents beriberi; and iron, which prevents anemia. And, to make it comparable to butter, margarine has been enriched with vitamin A, which is essential for growth, for maintaining healthy tissue, and which aids night vision.

The Recommended Dietary Allowances for the various minerals were established in 1980 by the Food and Nutrition Board, but some of these figures may be changing in the near future, according to Professor Beal. Calcium is one important mineral that has been under extensive investigation over the past few years. Many researchers have recommended a considerable increase in daily calcium intake by adult women to aid in the prevention of osteoporosis, or bone brittleness, which is the major cause of hip fractures. "The present recommendation is for 800 mg of dietary calcium a day," Professor Beal explains, "but this figure will probably go up to 1,000 mg. And for postmenopausal women, the recommendation by many researchers is for somewhere between 1,200 and 1,500 mg."

As with supplements in general, Professor Beal strongly urges that every effort be made to improve dietary intake to meet suggested requirements. "We need to understand that the body cannot fully utilize and absorb a single nutrient by itself. Nutrients as they are naturally present in our foods are bound to other nutrients which aid in absorption and utilization. The body cannot use calcium just by itself—other things have to be present in the G.I. tract so that it can be used by the body. Each nutrient has to be aided by other nutrients and enzymes to be picked up and transported to the intestinal wall—there has to be a carrier. In the circulation, again the nutrient has to be attached to something else in the blood to make it available to the body. When we take single mineral supplements, we disturb the balance of other minerals."

It is certainly possible to overindulge in mineral supplements. Presently, it is popular to take zinc supplements. But large amounts of zinc can cause heart disease by interfering with the body's use of copper, according to Dr. Walter Mertz of th U.S. Department of Agriculture. He states, "At a certain level, not overly high, zinc can interact with other essential trace elements, notably copper. You can produce a relative copper deficiency. Unfortunately, at present, it just happens to not be fashionable to swallow copper also." Professor Beal concurs that this "trendy" use of supplements is not wise. "We do not contribute to health by taking these random doses of single nutrients. Making improvements in our daily diet is what we need to aim for, unless a deficiency is diagnosed and a specific supplement medically prescribed."

The best calcium sources available to us are milk and milk products, canned sardines and salmon eaten with bones, dark green leafy vegetables, and dried peas and beans. Professor Beal suggests a variety of calcium-containing foods that can be combined to meet daily requirements. It is of special interest to note that skim milk contains more calcium than whole milk while being much lower in calories and fat.

Table 12.2 Sources of Calcium

Foods	Calcium Content
Whole milk, 1 cup	290 mg
Buttermilk, 1 cup	300 mg
Lowfat milk, 1 cup	350 mg
Skim milk powder, 1/4 cup	400 mg
Yogurt, lowfat, 1 cup	345-415 mg
Swiss cheese, 1 oz	260 mg
Cottage cheese, 1 cup	230 mg
Cheddar cheese, 1 oz	210 mg
Broccoli, 1 stalk cooked	160 mg
Mustard greens, 1 cup cooked	180 mg
Collard leaves, 1 cup cooked	360 mg
Okra, 1 cup cooked	150 mg
Sesame seed meal, 1/4 cup	270 mg
Tofu, 4 oz	150 mg
Soybeans, 1 cup cooked	130 mg

Note. From personal communication with Virginia Beal, PhD, University of Massachusetts.

Professor Beal feels that the pharmaceutical industry puts fears into people by making statements such as, "If you think your diet is not adequate, you better take this or that product." Most people don't know if their diets are adequate in all areas and begin to worry. "There is so much publicity about the horrible American diet, and I get quite provoked, because our diet is not horrible. We are not dying of malnutrition in this country. If anything should be of concern, it is being overnourished. We have a very good record in terms of longevity. We must be doing something right if people are living to be 70, 80, 90, or even 100 years old. In terms of general health in the older years, we are con-

cerned about heart disease, cancer, and stroke—these are the three major killers. Heart disease has been going down steadily for the last 20 years. You can find many reasons for this decrease depending on what your research interest is. We can say that eating less butter has contributed—except that many people who eat butter are also living perfectly healthy and long lives. You can say that it's because people are more exercise-oriented. Exercise certainly has been a factor. But chances are that there probably are 15 factors altogether in the causation of heart disease. The reason we are concerned about these three major diseases is because people in this country live long enough to develop them. In many populations, people die so much younger that these health problems don't have a chance to develop. We should appreciate the fact that the great variety of nutritious foods available to us is contributing to the longevity we enjoy in this country compared to other parts of the world."

vitamin Z

Professor Beal's most emphatic recommendation is that, especially at an older age, we keep vitamin Z in the diet. "I invented vitamin Z—it's the enjoyment vitamin. Nutritionists, dietitians, and physicians tend to tell people what they should or shouldn't eat. Instead, we should ask first which foods are important in that person's life and go from there. Foods have so many different meanings to people. There is so much ethnic influence, and it's interesting to look at why people like certain foods. Take the old favorite, chicken soup, which is known as the 'Jewish mother's penicillin.' But chicken soup, quite apart from being a Jewish favorite, has a lot of other things going for it. It smells good, tastes good, it's warm, and it goes down easily. And that immediately plugs in a strong factor for chicken soup in a sick child and will be imprinted as a favorite food. Each individual enjoys certain foods, and it's wrong to put a person on a standard diet that eliminates all these favorite foods. Let's look first at where enjoyment in eating comes from and then make adjustments in the form of as little change as possible. After all, these people have enjoyed a particular diet throughout life, and taking it away from them will make their lives much less enjoyable. Reducing diets are totally unsuccessful for these reasons—if we cut out all the foods we truly love, we end up being miserable. Let's enjoy foods in the later years rather than feeling that every bite of our favorite foods is doing us harm of one kind or another. Let's consume calories in moderation and keep good variety, including special treats, in our diets. And let's be wary of food quackery and new diet fads which promise instant weight loss, disease prevention, magic cures, and the fountain of youth. Our money is better spent on healthful, nutritious, and readily available foods from the supermarket."

epilogue

Many of you may already have successful programs in place, and I would love to hear from you. Sharing your experiences and making suggestions for additional resource materials, music, exercises, and activities your students enjoy would make an important contribution to developing more materials for all of us working in this field.

It has been a pleasure and privilege for me to write this book. It has helped me look at my work with renewed commitment and enthusiasm, and I sincerely hope that these materials will make a contribution to the health and wellness of our older population by encouraging well-prepared, enthusiastic fitness leadership. Make your program special. Do your work with an open mind and a sincere heart. Let your classes be a joyous experience, not only for your students, but also for yourself. Whatever is contained in this guide can come to life only through you, and I hope that your teaching will be special and rewarding.

appendix A
pulling it all together: sample lesson plans

Take another look at the "exercise pie," and use it as an approximate guide as you plan your classes:

1. *Warm-ups:* 5 to 10 min
2. *Exercises for specific muscle groups:* 15 min
3. *Endurance activities:* 20 min
4. *Tapering off:* 5 min
5. *Limbering, stretching:* 10 min
6. *Relaxation:* 5 min

Remember to keep exercises and activities well balanced. Keep changing body positions, alternate the use of muscle groups, and do something easy after more demanding sets of exercises. Avoid muscle soreness and fatigue by progressing slowly. Do a little more each time you meet, building up slowly to achieve a higher level of fitness. "Labor without weariness"—let this be your guide as you prepare each lesson.

Keep movements simple to ensure a feeling of success for everyone. Complete and correct movements at a reasonable pace are more beneficial for your seniors than many speedy repetitions. Keep to a reasonable number of repetitions of each exercise, changing to a new movement often but without rushing.

Participate in all activities you teach: Set an example and demonstrate correct movement. Be an educator: Explain while you demonstrate to help develop better understanding of the body in motion. Explain purpose and benefits of suggested exercises and activities, and encourage questions. Let everyone participate within individual limitations; there is no set expectation, no need to keep up with others, no reason to compete.

Stay enthusiastic and encouraging. Monitor your class, and stay sensitive to facial expressions and body language. They signal important positive and negative reactions.

At all times, stay concerned about everyone's safety and well-being. And, most importantly, make each class a time for feeling youthful and alive, for sharing in a different kind of "Happy Hour."

first lesson

Keep foremost in mind that the first class is an introduction to your program. Keep the atmosphere light and cheerful, making what may be a first exercise experience for many as enjoyable as possible. Be relaxed to help everyone else be comfortable. My suggestions can serve only as an approximate guide; make decisions based on what feels right, and stay flexible as the hour progresses. Use music selections that are no more than 3 minutes long.

Warm-up set #2: Reach and stretch Use moderately paced music for comfortable upper body stretching to feel tall and limber. Stretching helps to get in touch with how much stiffness there may be, and how good it feels to get some kinks out.

Warm-up set #3: Twist and limber Comfortably paced twisting movements are good for limbering waist and low back. Arm swinging helps increase blood circulation.

Warm-up set #5: Shoulder rolling Relaxed, graceful movements limber shoulders and stretch chest muscles and shoulder girdle. Leg movements lubricate knee joints. Use soft music.

Chair exercise set #9: Foot, ankle, and lower leg strength Focus on standing in good posture for these movements, which strengthen feet, ankles, and calf muscles.

Chair exercise set #10: Low back limbering, buttock muscles Involve large muscle groups in lower body with these swinging movements.

Chair exercise set #14: Leg strength Sit down for various leg movements to tone hip flexor and quadricep muscles and to work on more low back flexibility.

Put chairs away next.

Briefly discuss importance of endurance work for heart and lung efficiency and improved blood circulation, for feeling energetic, and for keeping bones strong.

Using brisk, well-paced music, take an energetic walk around the room, adding basic arm movements for upper body exercise. Walk with purpose and in proud posture.

Introduce wooden dowels, and bring the class together at one end of the room.

Endurance set #11: Walk with dowel Walk back and forth, practicing a number of the steps suggested to work on coordination and posture.

Endurance set #12: Walking with partner and dowel Repeat some of these patterns with a partner. Pair up by height.

Endurance set #24: Dowel catch in circle Bring everyone together into a circle and spend a few minutes with this activity to have fun and work on coordination and reaction time. Don't aim for perfection.

Endurance set #25: Partner stretching, share one dowel To cool down after this more active part of the class, spend a few minutes with stretching exercises. Demonstrate and explain movements.

Next, take carpet samples out for floor exercises. Explain first how to get down and back up from the floor safely, and practice together several times.

Floor-sitting exercise set #2: Hip joint limbering Spend a few minutes with these limbering exercises for hip joints and lower back.

Floor-sitting exercise set #3: Back and leg stretching Stretch hamstring and back muscles to relaxing music.

Partner exercise set #4: Waistline and trunk stretching Using partner's back for support, stretch slowly and breathe deeply. End with a wriggling back massage, and leave in high spirits.

second lesson

Dowel exercise set #1: Stretching with dowel Comfortable, relaxed bending and stretching movements limber waist, lower back, and trunk muscles. Use dowel for correct positioning.

Dowel exercise set #4: Leg kicking Warm up with brisk leg movements and work on coordination. Follow with walking briskly for a few minutes, dowel behind shoulder blades for posture awareness: chin up, chest out, stomach in.

Dowel exercise set #6: Knee-bending Lubricate knee joints, limber spine, strengthen quadriceps, and warm up all over with stretching and knee-bending.

Chair exercise set #16: Chair polka Choose a happy beat for a sitting polka. Introduce coordination movements that are not too confusing. These brisk arm and leg movements are tiring, in spite of the sitting position. Finish with tall stretching and deep breathing.

Chair exercise set #3: Shoulders and upper back
Stretch shoulder girdle, limber shoulder joints, and stretch spine.

Chair exercise set #7: Hands and wrists Use finger joints and wrists, and improve circulation in hands.

Chair exercise set #11: Standing to stretch Stretch long back muscles, shoulders, waistline, and leg muscles.

Next, put chairs away and start more active work: Without music, demonstrate and practice grapevine step together. Help those who have difficulty with this new step. Focus on relaxed movements.

Repeat these practices with a partner, moving from one end of room to the other, using music now.

Come together in a circle, hold hands, and practice as a group, going to the right, then to the left, coordinating leg movements.

With happy music, practice new walking patterns, going back and forth. Get everyone involved with hand clapping patterns, and work at coordinating arm movements with walking steps.

Abdominal exercise set #1: Back-lying abdominals
Demonstrate these exercises; then stand up to talk the group through this set. Observe, and make individual corrections when necessary.

Kneeling exercise set #1: Back limbering, buttock strengthening Introduce kneeling exercises, making sure that those with knee problems use very good padding. Demonstrate without music and don't rush these movements.

Floor exercise set #7: Waistline stretching Do various stretching movements in sitting position.

Front-lying exercise set #4: Low back/buttock strengthening Do various leg raising movements, and use good padding to protect pelvic area and rib cage.

Next, get up and form a circle, holding hands. Raise all arms high to inhale and stretch very tall; then bend knees, bring hands to floor, and exhale forcefully. Repeat several times.

Finish by "making sunshine," giving each other a happy back rub (Set #3, Ending a class), and leave feeling warm and relaxed.

third lesson

Warm-up set #1: Swimmers' warm-up Brisk upper body movements get blood circulating and warm up muscles.

Warm-up set #6: Arm, shoulder, and leg warm-up
Relaxed arm swinging. Limbers shoulders; knees become involved.

Warm-up set #9: Hip limbering Hip movements limber hip joints, lower back, and knees.

Warm-up set #10: More hip limbering Learn some new movements, and do grapevine step to right and left with music.

Next, *introduce beanbags* to start endurance activities.

Beanbag set #4: Tossing Each person has one beanbag and practices various tossing and catching movements with much bending to pick lost beanbags up. Now practice walking across room, tossing and catching while walking.

Endurance set #34: Tossing, group work Continue these activities, working as partners, with focus on agility, reaction time, and coordination.

Endurance set #35: Cooling down with partners
Practice standing and sitting movements with beanbag to slow down and work on flexibility.

Beanbag set #3: Finger exercises Everyone sits on floor with one beanbag for kneading and squeezing hand exercises.

Beanbag set #5: Sitting, stretching Stretch muscles in back of body with help of beanbag.

Introduce skipping: Demonstrate light, relaxed skipping, adding various arm movements for whole body involvement. Choose light, happy music to support this activity. Go back and forth across room, combining skipping and walking steps into fun patterns.

Endurance set #2: Walking patterns Form four groups, one for each corner, to walk diagonally across room. Alternate brisk, more demanding patterns with easy, fun steps. End with relaxed walking and arm swinging.

Chair exercise set #6: Coordination teasers Without music, work on coordination with these arm and leg movements. Demonstrate and explain, and have fun.

Chair exercise set #12: Thighs, hip flexors, and abdominals Introduce first three exercises and focus on correct sitting position. Alternate with stretching and forward-bending.

Chair exercise set #17: Stretching and bending Do some slow, relaxed bending and stretching with deep breathing to relax and feel loose and limber at the end of the class.

Finish with body wake-up, chair exercise set #1, spending the last few minutes with self-massage.

fourth lesson

Warm-up set #4: Arm crossing Arm swinging with leg involvement. Eliminate light jumping and coordination patterns.

Warm-up #8: Chest stretching Limber shoulders, and stretch chest and shoulder girdle.

Warm-up #11: Side-bending Do a progression of bending exercises. Start without music to become aware of the muscles involved; then add soft music.

Warm-up #4: Arm/leg coordination Demonstrate each step with arm movement, practice together, then repeat with music. Finish by walking around without losing pattern.

Endurance set #1: Practice prancing in erect posture, working feet and ankles. Add more energetic steps, lifting knees higher.

Introduce scarves: Each person has two scarves for energetic arm swinging while walking, skipping, or waltzing to happy music.

Repeat in rows of 6 or 8, coordinating swinging and leg movements in each group. Vary more demanding steps with easier ones.

Slow down, standing in place, and swing scarves with graceful, relaxed arm movements, choosing from the variety suggested. Keep leg muscles involved.

Partner exercise set #1: Abdominal strength Find a partner to give sit-ups a try. Strong ankle support is very helpful. Introduce the bent-knee sit-up, first progression, and the "lifeline" sit-up, trying five of each. Take turns.

Partner exercise set #3: Stretching Demonstrate again. Then observe and help where necessary.

Abdominal exercise set #2: Back-lying abdominals Make sure each person has a rug. Demonstrate and explain each exercise, and choose slow music.

Front-lying exercise set #1: Upper back, arms, shoulders These exercises are not easy; avoid too many repetitions. Relax and stretch, sitting back on heels, arms stretched long.

Back-lying exercise set #1: Hip and body raising Relax and stretch abdominal muscles; focus on controlled spine movements. Again, demonstrate and explain, and use relaxing music. Breathe deeply.

Ending a class, set #9: Come together to sit in a circle, legs crossed, for slow, relaxed neck movements with deep breathing.

Finish by sitting with legs straight and together. Stretch tall to inhale, and bend forward over relaxed legs to exhale. Repeat several times. Leave feeling well-exercised but relaxed.

fifth lesson

Warm-up set #20: Knee-bending Tall stretching alternates with half knee-bends and swinging movements for whole body warm-up and back limbering.

Warm-up set #15: Knee and leg lifting Alternate knee and leg lifting movements for lower body warm-up.

Warm-up set #7: Coordinated arm swinging Large arm movements increase heart rate. Add leg patterns after demonstrating, turning your back to the class. Practice without music first to keep confusion to a minimum; then repeat with music.

Endurance set #9: Grand march This takes some explanation and practice without music before putting it all together, marching to a steady beat next.

Endurance set #17: Polka Demonstrate a light, relaxed polka step. Finding the right music will make it easy for everyone to follow. Go back and forth for the length of your music selection, alternating easy steps with more vigorous ones. Arm movements add upper body exercise.

Endurance set #18: Polka with partners Continue to polka, holding hands with partner and coordinating feet. Combine walking with polkaing, and keep things uncomplicated as you introduce these movements.

Ending a class set #4: Partners, standing to stretch Take a short break from these endurance activities to stretch muscles in back of body with partner's help.

Endurance set #6: Handshake circle Bring everyone together in circle formation, staying with partner. Explain and practice this activity without music. Then add a happy tune and have everyone walk through this pattern with brisk steps.

Endurance set #8: Coordinated leg swinging in circle To finish the active time, stay in circle formation for leg swinging without music. Talk the group through some of the suggested movements so that everyone works together.

Introduce webbing bands in this lesson.

Endurance set #29: Floor-sitting in groups of five Each person should use carpet padding for group sit-ups and stretches. Again, demonstrate first; then work together to feel graceful while working abdominal muscles.

Webbing bands set #1: Standing to stretch Groups dissolve, and everyone gets up to stretch individually with one folded band. Twisting, bending, and stretching with the help of this hand equipment works on overall upper body flexibility.

Webbing set #4: Back-lying abdominals Explain and demonstrate clearly before having everyone try some of the easier abdominal exercises from this set. Then observe, and give individual help where needed.

Webbing set #3: Sitting stretches With feet anchored in loops of bands, spend a few minutes with leg and back stretching exercises. Roll bands up for storage.

Floor exercise set #1: Upper body strength If there is enough energy left, try a few of these body lifting exercises, slowly and with control, keeping to the easiest.

Back-lying exercise set #2: Low back and waist limbering Slow, relaxed movements limber lower back and waist. Stand up and talk the group through these exercises, using soft music to help everyone completely relax after a vigorous hour.

End with long, skinny stretching, inhaling deeply; then curl up into a tight ball and exhale. Repeat several times.

sixth lesson

Start this class with everyone walking in individual patterns, using all available space. Shake hands with others as you meet. Alternate walking with easy, relaxed skipping or polka steps. Spend three minutes, swinging arms as you walk and skip along.

Warm-up set #9: Hip limbering Knees, hips, and lower back limber up with these movements.

Warm-up set #18: Weight shifting When large leg muscles are used, body temperature rises quickly. Make sure legs are far enough apart for solid balance, knees directly over feet as weight shifts from one leg to the other.

Warm-up set #13: Forward and back bending Keep these movements relaxed, feeling like a ragdoll on forward bending, for overall limbering and back stretching.

Everyone takes a chair next.

Chair exercise set #15: Legs, feet, and fun Work on quick reactions, agility, and coordination. Choose just a few of the suggested movements, and combine them into a coherent sequence.

Chair exercise set #13: Abdominals and hip flexors Sit down for leg lifting and swinging to strengthen these important muscle groups. Keep to a reasonable number of repetitions, alternating the more demanding with easier ones.

Chair exercise set #5: Arm and back strength Take enough time to explain and demonstrate these exercises which require practice to be performed correctly. Make sure that all chairs have stoppers so that everyone is safe when trying push-ups. Finish with long back stretching to relax arms and shoulders.

Endurance set #21: Endurance work with chair support While chairs are handy, introduce some light jumping, holding on to chair back. Demonstrate, keeping steps feathery. Alternate light jumping with leg lifting or jogging in place.

Before moving chairs out of the way, spend a few minutes with stretching.

Introduce inner tubes in today's class.

Endurance set #30: Obstacle run Place tubes throughout room and run, staying light on feet. Find light music to keep a feathery feeling. Jump into and out of tubes occasionally, or take giant steps over tubes.

Endurance set #32: Tube competition Spend a few minutes with this fun activity, but observe your group to make sure that exertion is kept at a reasonable level.

Everyone takes one tube and a carpet square to cool down from these activities with a partner. Each pair uses two double-folded tubes for standing stretches, then to sit down for some sit-ups and more stretching. Put tubes aside.

Abdominal exercise set #5: Floor-sitting Demonstrate four exercises only, eliminating the more difficult ones.

Floor-sitting exercise set #4: Leg stretching Spend several minutes with forward-bending, tall stretching, and deep breathing. End by sitting with knees bent and open, soles of feet touching, and let upper body drop forward between legs, head hanging. Arms, shoulders, wrists, and hands are loose. Let everything feel limp.

seventh lesson

Warm-ups with scarves Start today's class with "flying colors." Each person holds two scarves for energetic arm swinging, arm crossing, and arm circling movements. Involve legs throughout.

Use scarves to add variety to side bending, twisting, and overall limbering exercises in standing position.

Return scarves to storage.

Warm-up set #16: Leg forward kicking Get legs moving with energetic kicking to peppy music. Those with balance problems should use chair support.

Introduce dumbbells today.

Dumbbells set #1: Upper body strength It is important to find just the right music to support these movements which should be performed slowly and with control. Alternate arm lifting with relaxed swinging, but grip the weights securely. Focus on deep breathing, and keep to a low number of repetitions of each exercise.

Walking with dumbbells: Move to one end of the room and add brisk walking to arm movements, staying with simple arm patterns. To be safe, stay far enough away from each other.

Return dumbbells to storage and take out dowels.

Endurance set #22: Serpentine run Form two single lines for this light running activity, placing dowels in two long rows on floor. Go back and forth several times.

Endurance set #23: Dowel obstacle course Practice light running and jumping patterns, being careful to clear each dowel. Give this activity enough time. No one should feel rushed while trying to coordinate these light jumps over all obstacles. Those with poor coordination need more time.

Endurance set #27: Partners share two dowels Cool down after these running and jumping activities with side bending, arm lifting, and swinging movements.

Endurance set #7: Snake dance This activity will take some time to explain, demonstrate, and then do. Plan on 10 minutes.

Ending a class set #3: Coordination walk Stay in circle formation and hold hands to learn this walking pattern. Talk the group through the changing steps, and explain the breakdown of a count of 8 into shorter sets.

Take rugs out, and join up with a partner.

Partner exercise set #2: Trunk raising Demonstrate these movements slowly and explain clearly, with emphasis on slow lifting movements rather than swinging trunk up. Don't use music, but talk and explain while everyone learns these new exercises. Give help where needed.

Kneeling set #3: Limbering and stretching Stretch tall to relax back muscles after these more demanding trunk raising exercises, and limber up waist with side bending. Keep these movements slow and relaxed, with soft music.

Abdominal exercise set #3: Back-lying abdominals Explain and demonstrate. Stand to talk group through these exercises. Focus on rhythmical breathing.

Back-lying exercise set #3: Low back stretching Comfortable curling exercises to stretch lower back. Stretch leg muscles which always tighten up after endurance activities.

Back-lying exercise set #4: Total body stretch To relaxing music, perform slow stretching and deep breathing exercises to end feeling very limber and relaxed. Stand to talk the class through these movements, keeping your voice soft and relaxing.

eighth lesson

Warm-up set #2: Reach and stretch To get in touch with your body, stretch tall to elongate waist, reach high to stretch rib cage.

Warm-up set #5: Shoulder rolling Everyone enjoys these relaxed limbering movements to soft music, stretching chest and shoulder girdle, limbering shoulder joints.

Warm-up #11: Side bending Slow, relaxed side bending and upper body circling for overall limbering, low back range of motion.

Bring out beanbags next.

Beanbag exercise set #2: Bending and stretching Involve leg muscles and knee joints, and work on coordination. Toss and catch beanbags, trying the "under-the-knee" and the "over-the-shoulder" tossing movements. There will be much moving around to retrieve stray beanbags.

Practice the "zipper opener" over both shoulders. Then walk around for a few minutes, tossing and catching beanbags.

Use dumbbells again today. Walk back and forth with various lifting and swinging movements while walking briskly. Music needs to be well-chosen and unrushed to allow for complete arm movements. Alternate more demanding movements with relaxed arm swinging.

Dumbbell exercise set #2: Upper body strength Repeat some exercises you introduced during the last class, and add some new ones. Focus on deep breathing, unrushed and complete arm movements. Demonstrate large front-to-back arm circling, and discuss importance of good range of motion in shoulder joints for daily activities and work. Return dumbbells to storage.

Endurance set #10: The Alley Cat This is easiest if you can find the Alley Cat music. Demonstrate first, practice briefly without music, and then have fun trying to work together with music.

Endurance set #14: Light hopping and kicking
Choose feathery music to help everyone stay light on their feet and keep exertion at a reasonable level. Instead of staying in place, move around with some of these movements.

Endurance set #19: Serpentine run Move to one end of the room and lead your class for light jogging in serpentine pattern. Be conscious of setting the pace. Those who get tired should walk briskly instead of continuing to jog.

Cool down with brisk walking and arm swinging, ending with slow, long steps and relaxed arm movements, deep breathing. Everyone takes a rug now for floor-sitting exercises.

Abdominal exercise set #4: Floor-sitting abdominals
Demonstrate and explain clearly the curling movement, keeping spine round and abdominals contracted. Alternate abdominal exercises with forward stretching to balance these movements.

Floor exercise set #6: Upper back and neck stretching Demonstrate correct positioning and form for slow, relaxed stretching. Try the "balance challenge," focusing on fun rather than perfection.

Ending a class set #15: Partners Sit across from a partner for some curling and stretching, combined with hugging by reaching for each other.

Ending a class set #10: Back-lying relaxation Conscious tensing and relaxing of individual muscle groups will help everyone feel relaxed at the end of this class. Rest for a minute, focus on deep breathing, and finish by stretching very tall, arms overhead, to go home well aligned and feeling trim.

These suggestions are intended only as a basic guide to help you prepare your classes for the first few weeks. There may be far too much material included in each lesson plan, but adjustments and changes are easy to make. Whatever develops during the course of the class hour, keep the basic progression of exercises and level of intensity in mind, and make your adjustments according to the group's ability.

Stay flexible. There is little value in rigidly adhering to your prepared materials, but much to gain from making adjustments to meet the needs of your class at any given time. Let your ultimate goal be to have a good time, move as much as is reasonable, and have participants leave feeling energized and well.

appendix B
suggested music

Ray Conniff/alone again—
Columbia #KC 31629

- "Candyman" for grapevine steps, alone or with partner; hip circling, foot steps with arm swinging.
- "Happiest Girl" for relaxed arm swinging, slow shoulder rolling.

Ray Conniff/world hits—
Columbia #CS 9300

- "Moscow Nights" for light jogging.
- "Greenfields" for relaxed head swinging and neck limbering.
- "Granada" for scarf swinging.

Ronnie Aldrich/melodies
from the classics—
Decca London #SP 44300

- "Adagio" and "La Mattinata" for relaxing.
- "Rondo Alla Turca" for walking with scarves or dowels.
- "Cavatina" for slow abdominals or sitting stretches.

music for a sunny Sunday—
Deutsche Grammophon #413 661

- Wonderful Viennese waltzes.

Chet Atkins, guitar/by special request—Victor #LSP 4254

- "I Saw the Light" for walking.
- "Difficult" for hip swinging and circling, leg rotation, travel twist.
- "Tiptoeing" for toe raises and leg lifting with chair support.
- "Everybody Does It" for upper body work with dumbbells and for back-lying exercises.
- Most other Chet Atkins records have a number of selections to use.

Floyd Cramer, piano/last date— RCA #AHL1-3487

- "Lover's Minuet" for weight shifting, knee lifting, chair support.
- "Never Ending Love" for soft arm swinging.
- "Morning Has Broken" for relaxed tall stretching, forward/back bending.

Bert Kaempfert and orchestra/ now—Decca #DL 75305

- "Put Your Hand" for leg kicking and for arm work with weights.
- "Red Sky at Morning" for relaxing.
- "Dream Baby" for arm swinging, arm circling, shoulder rolling.
- "Gray Eyes Make Me Blue" for skipping/polka combination.
- "Bell Bottoms" for jogging in place and knee lifting.
- Many of Bert Kaempfert's records contain good selections.

the magic organ/penny arcade— Ranwood #R-8100

- "Tacky" for hip swinging, kneebending, weight shift, twisting.
- "Road House" for steps in place with dowel or walking with dowel.
- "Magic Organ Polka" for walking and polka.
- "Penny Arcade" for swimmer's warm-up and chair polka.
- "Song Sung Blue" for slow stretching.
- "Beer Barrel Polka" for leg swinging and lifting, chair support.

exotic guitars— Ranwood #RLP 80002

- "Alley Cat."
- "Strangers on the Shore" for sitting stretches.
- 'Spanish Eyes" for kneeling exercises.
- "My Happiness" for kneebending and stretching.
- "Yellow Bird" for arm and leg raising, front-lying.

new christy minstrels/ramblin'— Columbia #CS 8855

- "Ramblin' " for walking with weights, walk and polka steps.
- "Mighty Mississippi" and "Ride, Ride, Ride" for light jogging.

sing along honky tonk— K-Tel Records NC-300

- "Japanese Sandman" for weight shifting.
- "Glow Worm" and "Ace in the Hole" for light jogging.

Herb Alpert/Alpert's ninth— AM Records #SP 4134

- "A Banda" for walking with arm movements.
- "Bud" for soft sidebending and twisting.

Raymond Lafevre and his orchestra/la la la— Four Corners #4250A

- "I Love You" for foot steps in place with arm swinging.
- "If I Only Had Time" for relaxing.
- "Delilah" for warm-ups and arm swinging.

Paul Mauriat and orchestra/ blooming hits— Philips PHS 600-248

- "Something Stupid" for soft bending and twisting, stretching.
- "Penny Lane" for walking.
- "This Is My Song" for relaxed head swinging.
- "Kind of Hush" for light jogging.
- "Puppet on a String" for brisk walking.
- "Love Is Blue" for relaxed polka steps, chair-sitting abdominals, kneebending/tall stretching.

Waldo de Los Rios/Mozartmania— United Artists UAS 5554

- "Mozart's 13th, Andante" for woodchopper and kneebending.
- "Menuetto" for knee drops or scissor kicks on back.
- "Rondo" for skipping and polka.
- "Mozart 21" for relaxing.
- "What Is Love" for stretching, bending, twisting.

hillside singers/I'd like to teach the world to sing— Metromedia #KMD 1051

- "Kum ba jah" for sitting stretches.
- "Amen" for relaxed arm swinging.

James Galway/songs of the seashore—RCA #ARL1-3534

- "Red Dragonfly" for twisting, bending, stretching.
- "Coconut Shell" for relaxed stretching.
- "The Moon on the Ruined Castle" and "Misty Moon Night" for relaxing.

James Galway/the pachabel canon—RCA #4063

- "Pachabel" for relaxing.

appendix C
suggested reading list

medical information

Guide to Fitness After 50
Raymond Harris, MD, and Lawrence Frankel (Eds.)
Plenum Press, New York, 1978

Presents basic and applied research data, authoritative advice, and tested techniques for professional workers and other individuals who want to learn more about physical exercise, fitness, and relaxation for older people.

Better Homes and Gardens After-40 Health and Medical Guide
Meredith Corporation, Des Moines, IA, 1980

Shares extensive medical information to provide better understanding of the structures and functions of body and mind and the process of health and disease.

The Best Years of Your Life
Miriam Stoppard, MD
Villard Books, New York, 1984

Comprehensive, fully illustrated guide to health and fitness after 50. Provides up-to-date thinking on aging and the latest medical findings on preventing or coping with common ailments.

Forever Fit—The Exercise Program for Staying Young
Morton D. Bogdonoff, MD
Little, Brown and Company, Boston, 1983

Includes suggestions for those who have heart ailments, back problems, and respiratory diseases. Directed at a general older readership. Author connected with the Duke University Center for the Study of Aging.

Stand Tall!—The Informed Woman's Guide to Osteoporosis
Morris Notelovitz, MD, and Marsha Ware
Triad Publishing, Gainesville, FL, 1982

Presents the latest findings of worldwide research on osteoporosis. Discusses comprehensive and in-depth options available for prevention, including information on exercise, nutrition, calcium supplements, and foods and drugs to avoid.

The Arthritis Helpbook
James Fries, MD, and Kate Lorig, RN
Addison-Wesley Publishing, Reading, MA, 1980

Guide to taking an active part in defeating arthritis with exercise, diet, and drugs. With contributions by members of the Stanford Arthritis Center.

The Body Machine
Christiaan Barnard, Consulting Editor
Crown Publishers, New York, 1981

Beautifully illustrated, comprehensive guide to the human body and its functions. Provides thorough knowledge of all body systems.

physiology- and exercise-related information

Exercise and Aging: The Scientific Basis
Everett L. Smith and Robert C. Serfass (Eds.)
Enslow Publishers, Hillside, NJ, 1981

Presents the value of exercise for improving the physical and mental well-being of the elderly. Identifies not only the structural but the functional aging characteristics of the major physical systems. Also supplies reliable information relative to current knowledge about the adaptation of these systems in response to regular physical activity. A well-edited, well-documented collection of papers presented at an annual meeting of the American College of Sports Medicine.

Physiology of Fitness
Brian J. Sharkey, PhD
Human Kinetics, Champaign, IL, 1984

Provides clear understanding of aerobic fitness, muscular fitness, the relationship between lifestyle and health, and the effects of fitness on weight control and overall health. Author is an exercise physiologist at the Human Performance Laboratory at the University of Montana.

Building Sound Bones and Muscles
Oliver Allen and the Editors of Time-Life Books
Library of Health/Time-Life Books, Alexandria, VA, 1981

Provides thorough understanding of the musculoskeletal system. Discusses joint and muscle function, back and foot problems, arthritis, bone health, sprains, strains, and fractures.

Be Alive as Long as You Live
Lawrence J. Frankel and Betty Byrd Richard
Lippincott & Crowell, New York, 1980

Includes simple, easy-to-learn exercises to help strengthen heart and lungs, tone muscles, and increase flexibility. A helpful guide for use at home by older persons or for conducting simple exercise programs for those who are physically more limited. Large print, fully illustrated.

The Simon and Schuster Handbook of Anatomy and Physiology
James Bevan, MD
Simon and Schuster, New York, 1978

"To visualize how the body works helps understand health and disease, prevention and treatment. When you appreciate structure you understand function."

This superbly illustrated handbook is enlightening and thorough in its presentation of structure and function—a wonderful reference for anyone interested in the human body.

Therapeutic Dance/Movement
Expressive Activities for Older Adults
Erna Caplow-Lindner, Leah Harpaz, and Sonya Samberg
Human Sciences Press, New York, 1979

Provides professionals with guidelines and specific material to conduct therapeutic movement sessions. Integrates creative and folk dance movements, yoga, and standard exercises especially adapted to the limited coordination and strength of the elderly.

Chair Exercise Manual
Eva Desca Garnet
Princeton Book Company, Princeton, NJ, 1982

Offers techniques, and chair exercises emerging from them, which have been tested by Ms. Garnet in classroom and hospital situations. For those with more limited physical ability. Available with audio-cassette.

nutrition information

The Lifelong Nutrition Guide
How to Eat for Health at Every Age and Stage in Life
Brian L.G. Morgan
Prentice-Hall, Englewood Cliffs, NJ, 1983

Advocates well-balanced, nutritious eating habits in a time of fad diets. Provides sound nutritional advice to live by at every age. Author is assistant professor of dentistry and nutrition at the Institute of Human Nutrition at the Columbia University College of Physicians and Surgeons in New York City.

Jane Brody's Nutrition Book
Jane Brody
W.W. Norton, New York, 1981

Helps those of us who are bewildered by conflicting nutrition information. Vital reading for everyone concerned with good eating and good health. Author has been a staff member of The New York Times since 1965 and has received numerous awards for excellence in science and medical reporting.

newsletters and magazines for staying up-to-date

Healthline is published monthly as a nonprofit public service by the Frederick Burke Foundation and San Francisco State University. Its contents are intended to educate readers about ways to help themselves avoid illness and to live longer, healthier lives.

To subscribe, contact:
Healthline
1320 Bayport Avenue
San Francisco, CA 94070

The Harvard Medical School Health Letter is published monthly by the Department of Continuing Education, Harvard Medical School, to provide accurate and timely health information for the general readership.

To subscribe, contact:
The Harvard Medical School Health Letter
P.O. Box 2438
Boulder, CO 80302

The Physician and Sports Medicine is a monthly journal serving the practicing physician's professional and personal interest in the medical aspects of sports, exercise, and fitness. Many of the articles are informative and helpful for those interested and teaching in the field of fitness.

To subscribe, contact:
Circulation Department
The Physician and Sports Medicine
4530 W. 77th Street
Minneapolis, MN 55435

American Health is published monthly to provide medical news, fitness, lifestyle, and nutrition information.

To subscribe, contact:
American Health Partners
80 Fifth Avenue
New York, NY 10001

The Tufts University Diet and Nutrition Letter is published monthly and always contains important and useful information to share with class members.

To subscribe, contact:
Tufts University Diet and Nutrition Letter
P.O. Box 34T
322 West 57th Street
New York, NY 10019

Nutrition & the M.D. is a monthly continuing education publication for physicians and nutritionists, but informative for general readership.

To subscribe, contact:
Nutrition & the M.D.
PM, Inc.
14349 Victory Blvd., #204
Van Nuys, CA 91401

index